BEAT
DEPRESSION
AND RECLAIM
YOUR LIFE

ALEXANDRA MASSEY

PUBLISHER'S WARNING: If you are currently
undergoing a course of prescribed medication for
depression, we strongly advise that you do not stop
taking it without first consulting your GP.

This edition first published in 2004 by
Virgin Books
Thames Wharf Studios
Rainville Rd
London W6 9HA

Copyright © Alexandra Massey, 2004

The right of Alexandra Massey to be identified as the Author
of the Work has been asserted by her in accordance with the
Copyright, Designs and Patents Act 1988.

ISBN 0-7535-0824-9

Designed by Smith and Gilmour, London

Printed and bound by Bath Press, CPI Group

CONTENTS

Foreword by Marjorie Wallace

In the twenty years that I have been campaigning to improve the lives of people with mental illness I have seen and heard some extremely distressing stories of mental torment and anguish. What keeps me going and gives me hope are the heart-warming stories of recovery like that of Alexandra who, through bravery and determination, are able to fight, if not always conquer, their inner demons and continue to live productive and fulfilling lives.

The World Health Organisation predicts that by 2020 depression will be the greatest burden of illness after heart disease. Such a grim prediction means depression is set to become more commonplace and there will be an increasing need for better therapies, services and medications.

I believe there is no single secret on how to beat depression that will work for everyone. Some people respond well to therapy, others to medication or a combination of both. Until we understand more about how the brain works there will always be an element of the unknown. We need to discover what changes may be happening and how those interact with the complex inner stresses, those profound emotional conflicts that drive and define our individual lives. People like Alexandra, who have survived their 'dark night of the soul', are able to offer hope and inspiration to others and we must rely upon them for sharing their triumphs and lessons.

I applaud Alexandra's self-help approach for its bravery and common-sense application. I am sure it will give inspiration to those able to take control of their lives to develop coping strategies and focus. It is with pleasure that I support this book and all those who take the journey with Alexandra to reclaim their lives.

Marjorie Wallace, Chief Executive of SANE
www.sane.org.uk

Introduction by Alexandra Massey

Depression affects most of us at some time in our lives. This book is for people who have suffered or are suffering a deep depression that is interfering with their lives and who cannot find a way out. It is for those who have contemplated suicide, felt wretched for months or years or who cannot see light at the end of the tunnel. It is for those who are struggling to find meaning and have failed. This book has been written to help you find your way out of depression. There are 10 suggestions to help you towards a life of fulfilment, contentment and joy, and a 14-day work plan that is intended to help you back on your feet. This book will offer hope to those who suffer every day and want positive change for themselves and those around them.

When I was severely depressed, I was sure that I did not want to resort to prescriptive drugs because, I was told (off the record) by a social worker, that if there was any problem with my son, as a single parent I was vulnerable to having my child removed from me. This scared me into going another route and searching for alternatives to beating depression without seeking help from medication.

The facilities that are needed to help people towards happier lives are limited on the NHS. Although counselling is available the waiting lists are long, and sometimes people have to wait many months before they can see someone. The problem is that if we need professional help for depression, we need it straight away. The most common method of treatment is to prescribe anti-depressants. These may offer a short-term solution, but the long-term effects can be counter-productive. Although there is a limited use for drugs, they may simply deal with the symptoms of depression by numbing our real feelings, and can create a long-term problem that becomes greater than the original symptoms due to drug dependence and the need to go through withdrawals. Recovery can be postponed by years.

This book tackles depression through a practical approach without medication. There are many excellent books devoted to the theory of overcoming depression, but this book does not delve too much into the theory. When we are depressed we do not always want to read into the mind of a theorist; we want to know what other sufferers have done to help themselves get better. This can help us to feel less isolated in our struggle to reclaim our life.

The book's title encompasses the phrase '... And Reclaim Your Life'. This refers to the point in our existence when we did have a complete life – because we were all born in one piece. As we have grown up, pieces have been taken from us. This book is about retrieving those stolen pieces and advocates recovery without the use of drugs. It discusses the routes to healing using inner reserve, community resources and clear-cut thinking.

How To Use This Book

The book is divided into two parts. The first part begins with some background information on depression, then presents the 10 suggestions in an easy-to-digest form that will help you through the darkest days. The second part is a day-by-day work plan that builds on the 10 suggestions, and this will really help you to begin fighting those awful, debilitating symptoms.

PART 1 ✳ THE 10 SUGGESTIONS

The 10 suggestions are divided into two sections:

'FIVE THINGS TO DO WHEN YOU ARE TOO DEPRESSED TO MOVE'

These are to be drawn upon when you are feeling so depressed that you cannot even be bothered to move. It is at this point that we need the most support but are probably in the least capable position to ask for it. When we're drowning in misery our assertiveness abandons us. We feel like a mound of sludge and become deaf to offers of help, misinterpreting the world and feeling isolated and lonely. We may become so hopeless that we feel suicidal.

But you are not the only one who feels like this. Take comfort in the actuality that there are millions of others who feel the same way. By undertaking some or all of the first five suggestions you will start to move away from the darkness and begin to grasp some hope. You will sense there is a way out even if you don't have all the answers. Recovery from depression is a slow but progressive journey. Take refuge in the first five suggestions and take them at your own pace.

'FIVE THINGS TO DO WHEN YOUR HEAD IS JUST ABOVE WATER'

These are for when the depression lifts just enough for you to put into place some ideas that you will be able to rely on if you go back into the depths of despair. They are the fast-track tools, intended to move you out of depression by helping you lift your denial. They are ideas that have been used by thousands of others to create new structures for dealing with their core problems. They are simple to comprehend but not necessarily easy to put into practice. They require the courage to change, and they are intended for when you have gained enough assurance through the first five suggestions. If you feel they ask too much of you, then stay in the first five suggestions until you are ready to make the next step. You will get to the point when you are frustrated with those first five suggestions enough to move on to the second five. Take them at your own pace and remember: easy does it.

PART 2 ✳✳ THE 14-DAY PLAN TO BEAT DEPRESSION

The second half of the book is a practical guide to put the 10 suggestions into practice. Sometimes, when you are severely depressed, it is helpful to follow a plan that has been successfully followed by others. Take on one task at a time, one day at a time.

This plan is laid out with examples and tasks that help put the suggestions into perspective. The tasks are set out in progression and are designed to help build a foundation of recovery. They have been designed so you can work towards achievable goals, and they give clear directions. The plan for taking action has been written to help deal with each tender, vulnerable part of you before moving onto the next.

The tasks do not need to be carried out across 14 consecutive days; indeed, they may be carried out over a number of weeks or months if it suits you. The plan requires a minimum of 14 days but it can be spread over an entire year, if that's what you need. The difference in time-span is entirely appropriate to your own history of your own depression. For those of you about to embark on the 14-day work plan, I would like to say that, although I do not know you personally, I know what you are going through, and wish you every success in the brave undertaking that you are about to begin. Stay with it, and be strong. There are many people going through what you are. You are not alone.

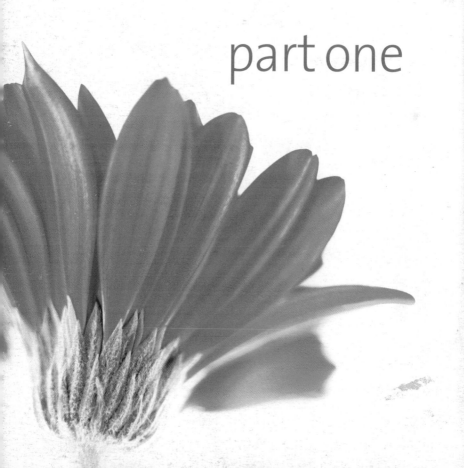

part one

What is Depression?

Depression is described in the dictionary as being 'low in spirit; downcast'. What it actually feels like is that a cloud of lead particles has settled on the soul. It is the heaviest weight we are ever going to feel. It is also the most stubborn of feelings and it can drive a person to despair. It sears our very essence and dirties our vision. It has the lightness of a gas but the weight of a concrete overcoat. It seeps into every crevice of our being.

When we are depressed we cannot be bothered with our own potential. We cannot lift our heads enough to see that we have true value in the world. We cannot give ourselves in close relationships because we become absent in the company of those we love. We care less about how we look, or else we overdo it when we go out to act as a mask to the world. We stumble through the day trying to find some meaning to the feelings that ravage us. We lose our motivation to pursue our true vocation and, in so doing, compromise our soul.

We feel like victims – buffeted by the rough winds of life. We cannot grasp onto anything that is solid in order to pull ourselves out of the storm. Either we see nothing but unfairness or we stoop to self-loathing and believe we deserve nothing better. We lose our sense of reason and we are unable to take an objective view on our circumstances and address what is fact and what is fiction.

And don't be fooled by those people who are deemed a 'success'. Many 'successful' people are on the run – running away from their own depression and trying to escape the darkness by making enough money or becoming so well known that the trappings of fame will cushion them from their distress. But the pain pursues them with inches to spare. The faster they run, the faster it runs. There is the old adage: 'When I get there, then I will be happy.' This thinking is a one-way track to disaster as, most often, we never arrive.

The problem with depression is that it does not allow us to stand still. We either get worse or we get better. One common symptom of depression is mood swings. We can go from feeling ecstatic to feeling suicidal in minutes. We are used to the highs and lows; we thrive on them to give meaning to the day. But this thinking exacerbates the depression by keeping us in a state of anxiety. When the process of recovery from depression begins, it can seem as though nothing is happening, but this may be because we have stopped the backward drag.

The fastest route to recovery is the hardest route. It involves dedication and exertion without props. It involves giving up and letting go. It requires us to acknowledge we have hit rock bottom. There are many ways to tackle depression and to help us move forward, but the most powerful approach is to turn around and face it head on. This will be the beginning of a change that will resonate for the rest of your life. You will look back and be excited about hitting this point. I look back and see that I would never have reached this point of restoration, excitement, hope, strength and joy had I not hit that point of no return. Restoration is available to anyone who embarks upon tackling depression through the suggestions in this book.

SOME SYMPTOMS OF DEPRESSION:

- Overwhelming tiredness
- Insomnia
- Self-loathing
- Rage
- Immense sadness
- Inability to do anything worthwhile
- Feeling dead
- Feeling stuck
- Feeling isolated
- Harming ourselves
- Feeling lonely
- Thoughts of suicide
- Not caring whether others like us or not
- Having no feelings – numbed
- Eating junk
- Smoking
- Sabotaging friendships
- Behaving violently
- Stealing
- Drug and alcohol abuse
- Gambling to excess
- Being obsessive about sex
- Losing all interest in sex
- Abusing children
- Compulsively cleaning

WHY ARE WE DEPRESSED?

The very word 'de-pressed' suggests that something is being pushed down. We are depressed because we have pushed down emotions that we cannot allow to come to the surface. We constantly experience a range of emotions; how we handle them determines the level of our mental health. If we feel angry but don't express that anger in a healthy way, we will either act it out in ways that are detrimental to us, or we will ignore it and push it down. If we feel sorrow but don't let it out, we hold back the tears until they are too 'pressed down' to be released. We all face adversity in our lives, yet how we respond to it is a direct response to the way we have been taught to react.

Most causes of depression are seated in the past. Research has shown that our personalities are moulded in the first six years of our lives and it is the quality of the care we receive in our early years that makes us what we are. It also dominates our choice of friends and lovers, shapes our interests, determines our careers and even changes our brain patterns and our body chemistry. It can also trigger mental illness, including depression and/or criminal behaviour later on in life.

When our life is wonderful, we don't question the way we tick. But when we hit a bad patch, if we don't have a compassionate, in-built method of dealing with trauma we can easily fall into a depressive state. Many scenarios can push us into despair when we don't have tools for counselling ourselves. Below are some common examples.

We have lost someone close to us
We can become depressed if someone we love has died. We can also become depressed if a close relationship has finished. In both cases the process we go through is similar (although highly personal).

We feel we have no control

We can become depressed if we are trying to control other people. Attempting to change another person only leads to frustration and disappointment, because we can never really have that power. This can occur in our intimate relationships, at work, with our children, in dealing with our parents or with friends. This is the unexpressed frustration and disappointment at others not behaving as we want them to.

Incapacity

Depression can set in if our body has let us down, through illness or incapacity. Many people who find themselves physically disabled become depressed because they cannot function like everyone else. This is also prevalent in elderly people whose physical bodies cannot move them around as they used to. Feeling physically helpless can be a major trigger of depression and hopelessness.

We are in a dead-end relationship

We may be in a relationship that we simply can't see a way out of. We feel trapped by circumstances and have fallen into the belief that we cannot move away from this dead-end place because we have no money, we have children to think of, or we simply would not be able to cope on our own. We feel that the relationship is the root cause of all our misery, yet we are stuck.

We feel powerless

We find ourselves depressed when we feel powerless or victims of circumstance. We are allowing someone else to dictate to us as if we were children. We may feel bullied and violated by another and feel that we are in a hopeless situation.

We are broke

There is nothing like struggling financially to feed our depression through feelings of anger and frustration, especially if we are powerless over our circumstances. If we have no way out we turn the feelings inwards and blame ourselves until we are full of shame and end up treating ourselves, and those around us, badly.

Post-natal depression

If someone is prone to depression, giving birth can trigger off a chronic bout. There is a lot of conjecture about why women become depressed after having given birth. Reams of medical papers are devoted to the theorising of post-natal depression and the role that hormonal change plays. However, there are some very simple explanations for it: being physically shattered; the overwhelming responsibility of caring for the baby; a feeling of isolation at home with our partner having returned to work, and maybe giving up our own job with all its support system. When we are depressed the last thing we want is to have to take care of a new baby, regardless of how much we adore it, but we feel we have no choice.

Retirement

Just sitting still with ourselves can be a traumatic experience if we've spent years being busy. Whatever we have been running from catches up with us when we stop. We are not experienced in sitting still and taking time to do what we want. We also give up the power and the glory of being needed and fulfilled in our previous role. Once we are retired, it can seem like our raison d'être has gone.

We are competing with everyone

The very nature of the 'civilised' world lends itself to many people feeling like a failure. In our better/best world, it is not hard to feel that we will never be good enough. We are constantly bombarded with ideals, images and stories about how we should live our lives. Icons are held up as examples of what we should achieve. Tales of others' perfect lives come at us every way we turn and it takes a strong character not to buy into these fantasies of what we need to buy/earn/sell in order to achieve happiness.

We have lost our childhood

For some of us, none of the above had to happen for us to feel depressed. We have always felt depressed and we don't really know what it's like not to feel that way. This is because we didn't have the childhood we were entitled to. The childhood we are entitled to is one that is full of fun and happiness; where we feel safe and warm knowing that, however naughty we are, we are still cherished. We should be fed and washed, be able to sleep soundly, and be nurtured and guided through life's lessons. If we are disciplined, it should be in a way that feels firm but fair.

Those of us who did not experience this may have grown up feeling isolated and uneasy with others, especially authority figures. We constantly seek approval and have lost our identity in the process. We get guilt feelings for standing up for ourselves and we put others before ourselves. We fear criticism and take it as a threat. We feel victimised and are attracted by this weakness in others. We judge ourselves harshly and have very low self-esteem. We have become dependent personalities who are terrified of abandonment and willing to do anything to hold on to a relationship.

GRIEVING FOR OUR LOSS

All of the above scenarios are about people having lost something and being unable to process it. Depression happens when we are stuck in this process. We may sit in the denial because we do not want to cry out the pain. We may push our anger down and be determined that we have no feelings. We may feel too guilty and believe we don't deserve to heal.

Even if we do not feel as though we lost our childhood, and are depressed for other reasons, how we deal with life's more difficult challenges – such as those listed above – is directly related to how we learned to deal with them as children. Negative influences from our past hinder our ability to function competently in the adult world and can lead to periods of depression and mental illness. People who do not deal with their unremitting depression can run the risk of ending up in prison, a mental institution or even dead. But there is hope for everyone to recover and many of us have recovered.

THE GRIEF PROCESS

All of these scenarios have one common factor – the natural cycle of the grief process has been hindered. We become depressed when we get stuck in the natural human evolution that we all experience. There is a natural ebb and flow of life and we all progress through it in a similar, albeit very personal, way. When we experience loss or trauma, we psychologically go through a sequence of transformations that assists us to cope with the loss.

Below is an illustration of the grief process:

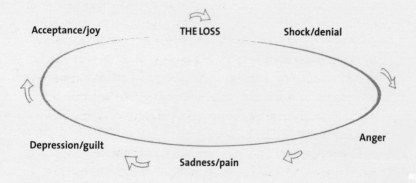

Grief is the normal but highly personal response to loss.
The grief process consists of a series of emotions that includes
shock, denial, pain and acceptance. Although depression is
a part of the grief process, we will not become stuck in it if
we are naturally progressing through the process. We become
depressed when we have stopped expressing the anger or
sadness of the grief process. These are the two most difficult
emotions to release. The irony is, we may have to go back
through the whole grief process again in order to shift
ourselves out of feeling depressed.

Loss on a large scale would include the death of someone
close to us. Losing someone propels us into a world of grieving
that takes us away from the normal bustle of life. First we go
into shock and cannot believe what has happened. We deny the
truth of it. We think there has been an error or that something
will change and bring that person back. We may renounce the
realism, hoping that we may be able to do something that will
reunite us with that person. Over time, the reality comes into
focus and we start to realise that the loss has actually happened.

We then go into a state of anger, blame, rage and frustration, wanting to blame others for not doing enough or even
blaming the person who has died for abandoning us. Once the
bulk of the anger has been vocalised, the sadness sets in and
it is time to cry for our loss. With this sadness may come hopelessness that the crying will never stop. Sadness comes and
goes and is intermingled with depression and guilt as we
realise that it wasn't us that died, that there is nothing we can
do about our loss, or that we cannot be happy again without
the person we have lost. This depression is a 'healthy depression' – a part of the natural grief process that takes us towards
acceptance of our loss. It is the final stage of the saying good-
bye to who/what we have lost, so we can come to terms with
how our situation has changed.

Eventually, when enough pain has been dispersed, we start
to believe we will make it through the darkness. The healing

that has taken place leaves us feeling lighter, and we move towards a sense of peace, acceptance and even – at a later date – joy once more. This is the natural process of grief that affects us all at some point in our lives. This process takes place not only when we have lost someone but also when we perceive that we have lost something – for example, through divorce, when our children leave home, when we have been made redundant, or when someone breaks off a friendship. One of the most prevailing losses for us that we don't often recognise is the loss of dignity, of personal power and, more often than not, our childhood. All these losses mount up.

If we do not go through the natural grief process we become stuck. The natural process is halted, the feelings are pushed down and we become depressed. If we are depressed, we must look at what we have lost but have not grieved over. This is a tremendous tool in helping us to reclaim our lives.

We may sit in the denial because we do not want to go through the pain. We may push our anger down and be determined that we have no feelings. Inside, we may feel guilty and believe we don't deserve to heal. Sometimes, though, those feelings may well up and be too strong for us to ignore.

The three main themes that emerge from this section and, indeed, that run through this book, are that we need to:
• unravel what belongs in our past
• understand what is accurate in the present
• grieve for what we have lost

These three concepts will give us the freedom to move forward, break the cycle of depression and lead us towards a more fulfilling life – which is our true birthright.

A WORD ABOUT DENIAL

Many people deny they are depressed. It's not that they deliberately lie to anyone; it's that they have to lie to themselves to keep going. Denial may seem from the outside like an ignorant state in which to live, but it is a very practical way of keeping a problem at bay. Denial is a form of survival. People who are denying their own depression need to be left alone until they are ready to come out of hiding on their own terms.

Many addictions are created to assist the individual to deny his/her problems. Although this may seem self-destructive, it has to be recognised that the addiction is, conversely, a form of survival. It is about surviving the depression by burying the painful feelings that go with being chronically depressed. For many people, the pain of addiction is not as great as the pain of depression.

RECOVERY VERSUS MEDICATION

The two options open to someone who is depressed are to face the depression head on and move into recovery or to 'medicate' the feelings to avoid the anguish that accompanies depression. Either way is gruelling. We either move forward or we move backward. We do not stay static. For the purpose of this book, we use the term 'medication' to describe anything that is used to avoid feelings. Medicating feelings can include excesses of the following: drugs, alcohol, nicotine, shopping, gambling, working, sex, eating, not eating, exercising, helping others, being perfect, judging others.

Facing the depression with a view to conquering it can be the hardest option. Medicating feelings is a way of not allowing ourselves to become overwhelmed with grief and pain. But we can face serious problems when the behaviour that serves to medicate depression becomes troublesome in its own right. If the drugs used to medicate depression force us to lose our job, or damage our family, relationships, friends etc., then we have another problem to address. It is at this point that either our denial lifts or we medicate further. I repeat: there is no static point – it moves forward or it moves backward.

We stop denying our problems when we feel strong enough to start dealing with them. When the denial lifts it can be very painful, but the human mind will not lift its own denial if it is not strong enough to cope with what it is trying to deny. The deeper the depression, the stronger the denial.

One thing we do not need is self-reproach for not having faced up to our problems sooner. The quicker we recognise that our denial has done us a great service, the better we will feel about moving forward. There is no point in pushing us when we are in denial. Denial is all-powerful and if there is a power-struggle taking place between our denial and someone who wants us to change, our denial will win. It is the 'mother of all saviours' and will prevent us from cracking up for as long as we need it.

When we medicate our emotions, we medicate everything. We cannot, unfortunately, just medicate our negative feelings and leave ourselves with a supply of good feelings. In medicating our depression we also medicate the ability to feel happy, joyful, excited and alive. It's all or nothing. I firmly believe that medicating anything medicates everything. This is where our denial will help. It will assist us to slow down the medication of our feelings, as and when we are ready. If someone badgers us to stop smoking, we can explain the options: 'I'll smoke thirty cigarettes a day or I'll drink a bottle of vodka a day and smoke twenty cigarettes a day. You choose!' This is the reality of confronting depression. We cannot put everything down in one go. It is a journey and, when we feel better about ourselves, we will harm ourselves less.

For the purpose of this book, I am going to assume that you are ready to start on that journey and face some of your problems. This often happens when all else has been tried and has failed. There is no need to address the denial, as this will have

begun to lift. Remember: denying your depression and
the pain that goes with it will lift and return. Recovery from
depression is like peeling layers of an onion. We peel one layer,
then, when we are ready, we will go on to the next. The denial
will help us pace ourselves until we are ready to deal with
the next layer.

MILESTONES

It is important to know what good things to expect when
you embark on this journey. For many of us, the goal is simply
to beat depression, but this can encompass many unknown
roads. For this reason, here is an outline of some of the mile-
stones that you will reach if you follow the suggestions and
the work plan.

- You can make mistakes and yet feel liberated from constant
  self-criticism
- Accept that your feelings are OK; they are not wrong or right,
  they are feelings
- There is no shame in struggling; you can release yourself from
  the pursuit of perfection
- It is OK to be honest about yourself; constantly lying is too
  complicated and exhausting
- You are entitled to want things
- Fear is a consequence of self-judgement; as you judge yourself less,
  so your fear will diminish
- Self-protection comes at a price; when you stop denying your pain,
  you open yourself up to the gifts of recovery
- You can laugh, play and have fun
- You can learn to take responsibility for your actions; this will help
  you regain your power
- You will need less 'things' from the world because you feel less
  pain and therefore need to medicate yourself less
- You will feel more accepted by others and start to enjoy the
  fruits of intimacy

The ideas formulated in the book serve to address all the different areas of life in which we cannot find immediate clarity while we are dogged with depression. They are not rules or commands but ideas for you to work with in the way that is best for you. Take what you like and leave the rest.

The 10
Suggestions

The suggestions do not need to be undertaken in order. They can each be taken up when they feel right for you. When you read a suggestion and it feels right, this could indicate that it is a good thing to do for yourself at that moment. With some of the suggestions, you may not feel safe in undertaking the advice and, for other parts, you may have to employ some 'blind faith'. These suggestions have worked for many people – myself included – and I'm grateful for all the wisdom I have received throughout my recovery from depression.

Five Things To Do When You Are Too Depressed To Move

1 SURRENDER

When you are in a full depression, there is really no point in trying to fight it. It is like riding a bicycle with a flat tyre. We keep getting off and pumping it up only to find that the tyre is flat once more minutes later. We are better off just accepting the status quo instead of fighting a battle we can't win. The harsh words we tell ourselves are akin to falsely pumping up that tyre again, only to feel deflated soon after. 'What's wrong with you?' – 'Pull yourself together, you idiot!' – 'You're a useless piece of shit!' – are admonishments that won't help. At times like this, just stop, breathe out and notice the release of tension in your stomach. Accept the depression for that moment. Know that you are depressed and, just for that moment, are completely powerless to change it.

This acceptance will bring you a sense of relief. It will calm you down in the knowledge that you don't have to sort it out there and then. You can just relax and sit with the feeling of being depressed. It is not self-indulgent; it is honest. You are entitled to feel depressed if that is how you feel. You can still function and be depressed. Being depressed does not mean you are going to die; it means you feel depressed. You can cope with that for one day at a time, one hour at a time, one minute at a time. You are not a freak, you are not unnatural, you are not worthless – you are simply depressed.

You are better off surrendering to your depression than trying to fight it. Like pushing wet sand, the more you push, the harder it gets. By surrendering you are putting your arms in the air and saying just that: 'I surrender.' Go on – try it. Just do it. You will feel the difference as you do it and you will feel some acceptance of your current state.

HOW TO SURRENDER

You must prepare well for this. You need time to yourself. It does not need to be all day but it needs to be at least one hour a day. However, the more time you get to yourself the better. You don't have to be on your own but you need to have little or no responsibility during your hour. Once this is organised, you must become aware of your duties for the week and cut them down to the bare minimum. If you have a job, take time off. If you have children, organise your routine as best you can to get as much time to yourself. You may feel that this is too much bother but also bear in mind how long you have been depressed and ask yourself how much longer you want to stay depressed.

At some point you have to surrender to the fact that you are suffering from depression and that you feel powerless over it. You have tried everything to change the way you feel and little has worked. For now, just admit that you are powerless over your depression – submit to your feelings.

It is vital for your recovery that you completely indulge in your feelings so that you feel saturated. This is because you have never allowed yourself to totally experience the despair and hopelessness that comes with depression. This is the goal of surrendering. We usually judge ourselves harshly for our state of mind, but this is the time for you to accept yours. This may be the most difficult part of beating depression because you have probably never allowed yourself to completely indulge in your despair. Stick with the simplicity of allowing yourself this time out.

EVERY DAY, DO AT LEAST SOME OF THE FOLLOWING:

- Sink into your depression
- Let go of trying to control your feelings
- Stop trying not to be depressed
- Don't soldier on any more
- Look down towards the floor and feel the weight on your shoulders
- Feel the despair and hopelessness
- Feel the unfairness and self-pity
- If tears rise to the surface, let them out
- Ask no questions
- Indulge in your melancholy – you have permission to do so
- Feel the anger if it rises to the surface
- Let out your anger if it feels right
- Take time off – get a sick note
- Concentrate on you and no one else
- Stay in bed, damn the world
- Reel with the self-admission that you are depressed
- Make no big decisions
- Abdicate as much responsibility as you can
- Shelve your projects
- Abandon your duties
- Suspend self-criticism for surrendering

Don't move on to the next suggestion until this period has finished. Put this book away, except to re-read the first suggestion. It is now time to completely let go. Don't be afraid of what might happen; you won't lose any more control than you have lost already. Good things will come from this stage. If you feel worse than you have ever felt before this is because the feelings that you have been running from are surfacing. But it is more exhausting to be constantly running than it is to STOP, turn around and face what you have been running from. You use up far more energy running away than turning around to face the unknown. This is because you have had to contend with the exhaustion of running plus the fear of the unknown!

When I had a breakdown caused by depression, it was the running away from the problem and the feeling scared of accepting that I was depressed that wore me down. Once I had begun to accept that I was depressed, I stopped betraying myself and sought help. This was the beginning of my road to recovery.

While you undertake these tasks, you may get a sense that your depression is not as great as you thought. It's the pushing away from the depression that can make it seem overwhelming. As in so many areas of life, when we don't face what we are afraid of, whatever is tormenting us can seem so much bigger than it really is. The only way to learn this lesson is to face the threat. Unfortunately, no one can do this for us. We have to do it ourselves.

However, the good news is that each time you face your worst fear, you will grow in stamina to do it again and your courage will increase. Depression can feel like a big, black, bottomless pit. The reality is, however, that it is your fear that creates the black hole, not the depression itself. As your recovery continues, you will begin to notice a foundation to the black pit; then the pit will become more shallow; finally, you may forget there was ever a black pit there at all.

2 ONLY DO THE NECESSARY

Don't do anything that you don't need to. Trying to perform when you feel depressed only compounds the message that there is something wrong with you. This is because you are trying to do things that, for the moment, are out of your reach. There is no point in competing with others at this time. Conserve your energy and, if you have the luxury of time, take yourself to bed or somewhere safe, and withdraw from the world.

There is no perfect time in the future to begin your recovery from depression; the time is right now. There is no point in obeying the rules of others and carrying on as if you are feeling 'fine'. Some time ago, when I was asked how I was and I answered 'fine', I was told it meant 'Frightened, Insecure, Neurotic and Emotional'! There is some truth in this because we all say 'fine' when we mean 'I feel like shit and I want to go to bed and hide from the world for a week.' It is time to be honest with yourself, put yourself first, and give yourself permission to take time out from trying to please others. Drop the responsibilities that do not matter. Those that do matter include caring for children, keeping yourself fed, warm and safe, and working to bring in just enough income to make do. Other than that, there are few responsibilities that you need to take on.

If you are thinking that this suggestion is not for you, then ask yourself this question: 'Who am I competing against?' If you are not willing to slow down your workload and minimise your commitments so that you get the rest and recuperation you need to beat depression, then you are faced with a chronic spiral of decreasing energy that will only leave you feeling more helpless and hopeless.

This is the madness of depression; we know we need to slow down and move towards helping ourselves, but we fear that we will never get going again if we stop. We are scared that if we stop being as busy as we are, then our pain will overwhelm us. But remember: your denial will only lift to present you with as much as you can manage at any one time. It is now that you need to employ some of that 'blind faith' I mentioned earlier.

We can find a way of getting time to ourselves, even if it means cancelling other priorities and diving under the covers. If you are frightened of coming to a complete stop, then achieve just one thing in your day and celebrate it at the end of each day – even if it is something as simple as making your bed. You will always feel better for it.

3 WRITE ABOUT YOUR DEPRESSION OR MAKE A TAPE

When you are under the oppressive weight of depression, write about it. Writing down the way you feel and what you think is comforting and will give you a sense of someone listening to you. Write the words as they flow from your heart to your fingers and allow them to spill out onto the page. This small achievement is enough to make a difference. It will help you to feel a little comfort when all else seems lost.

Having a beautiful journal to hand in which you can write helps you feel special because your words are being cherished. Writing when you need to can sometimes lead you to the reasons you feel depressed. As you write, let the words drop out of you as they come. Don't alter them to make more sense or to try to make them say what you think they should say. Simply let them be, with no judgement. Then re-read them and notice the feelings that appear in you. Don't judge the feelings but simply allow them to pass.

You can also use audio or videotape. Set up a machine into which you can talk. Speak as if you are talking to someone you can trust with all your secrets. As you talk, get to the bottom of how you are feeling. Allow yourself as much time as you need. Any machine that will play back what you have said is good enough – a Dictaphone is perfect. Once you have said all you want to say, play it back to yourself. You will be surprised at the results.

While you are doing this, begin to identify what makes you feel 'guilt' and what makes you feel 'shame'. These are two common themes we encompass if we are depressed.

Guilt is when we feel bad about 'what we have done'. Guilt lets us know there is something we need to address. It indicates that there is something about the way we have behaved that has had a negative effect on others. Staying stuck in the guilt keeps us from our sadness and we feel apart from others. Know that there is something we can 'do' to address our guilt.

Shame is when we feel bad about 'who we are'. We feel the core of us is bad but we cannot put our finger on why we feel like this. We feel shame for not being good enough, for letting others down, for needing others, for not taking care of our responsibilities. At its worst, shame tells us that we don't deserve to be alive.

When you have said everything you want to say at that moment, you will most likely realise that it wasn't as much as you thought it was going to be. The central point of your depression can often be summarised in a paragraph. It is surprising how simple the problem seems when you play it back. In listening to yourself, solutions will come to you. You will gain a sense of being heard, and this will help relieve the immensity of the despair for a little while.

❋ ❋ ❋

4 GET ANGRY / CRY

Depression holds down stuck feelings. Either you feel that you don't want to face those feelings or can't face them. Why? Because you think it would be too painful, and if you start to cry or get angry, you will never stop – and you don't want to feel out of control. The feelings may be so painful that staying depressed is preferable.

However, you have a tremendous inner reserve. Your spirit will not allow you to lose control. You will only release the feelings that you can handle. If you begin to cry, you will stop when your essence has had enough. If you let out the rage, you will become exhausted before you lose control. You will only be given what you can handle. You will only receive what you can manage. Your mind will only expend what it deems safe to expend. You will only be given what you feel is safe to let out. This is the natural human evolution. You have to trust yourself and push forward, because the central pivot to beating depression is to release those feelings. One person I counselled told me, 'When I was going through the mill, I had great concerns that I was in fact going mad and that serious damage would be done to my brain. Crazy, I know. However, I was told and I learned that this simply would not happen, as exhaustion would set in well beforehand.'

To help yourself get hold of the sadness or rage, imagine the feeling as you see it. What colour is it? Where does it sit in your body? What shape is it? I had always seen my sadness and rage as a solid grey concrete block that sat on the top of my chest. The effect it had on me was to drain me, pull me down, and leave me feeling listless, heavy and hopeless, because it seemed an impossible weight to carry. By seeing the feeling, you will start to see it as it is – a finite sensation that can be dealt with – not an unidentified object that you are unable to cope with. As you cry or rage, the enormity of the feelings will subside.

LETTING OUT THE ANGER

Anger that is not dealt with in childhood can develop into depression in adulthood. It can also develop into abuse of self and others, which leads to mayhem. I believe that behind every man and woman in jail for violent behaviour lies a part of them that is in deep pain. Childhood abuse creates abusive adults. Unexpressed anger can be very dangerous – to both ourselves and others – as the anger that is suppressed comes out as rage. We have to move on from our childhood rage in order to develop into competent and happy adults, but this is not easy.

Many of us deny that we are angry but, if we are depressed, then we have hidden our anger. We are not encouraged to express this emotion – especially as children – and we are not taught how to release it. But every one of us is angry about something, and unchecked anger can lead us into situations we would choose not to be in if we thought about them rationally. If we are angry and do not deal with that anger, it will land on the top of the angry heap inside us. It doesn't go away; it just accumulates.

HERE IS A CHECKLIST FOR HIDDEN ANGER:

- Chronic pain in the neck or jaw
- Sarcasm
- Ironic humour
- Boredom, apathy, disinterest
- Nightmares
- Smiling when you don't want to
- Controlling your voice
- Grinding your teeth at night
- Becoming irritated at irrelevant things
- Body tics or spasmodic movements that you are unaware of
- Stomach ulcers
- Constant cheerfulness and 'grin and bear it' attitude
- Refusing eye contact
- Clenching a thumb in a fist
- Over-politeness
- Not sleeping or sleeping too much
- Frustration at everything around you
- A feeling of one's life not being good enough

If you don't recognise any of these signals in yourself, ask people close to you if they recognise any of them. Ask them how they can tell when you are upset about something. Just hear their response without sinking into a pit of shame. Take it as good information. It is normal to deny that we are angry because it's the way our society is. When someone is angry, others often look at them and say, 'Ooh, what's wrong with her?' It isn't generally accepted that releasing anger is a path to freedom. But it is. So you must find yours. At this point you have to take it in blind faith that if you are depressed you will have repressed anger.

Take an hour aside for yourself and sit somewhere quiet and safe. Begin to write about what angers you. Make a list of at least ten things – you will begin to see a common theme. Whatever your common theme is, allow yourself to indulge in the fury that accompanies your list. My lists usually encircle one main problem in my life. The ten things on your list will guide you towards your object of vehemence. Forget yourself as the nice, polite grown-up and see yourself as a screaming unreasonable toddler who has had enough.

If you need to take action to dispel the anger, thump the pillow, run it out, throw rocks in the sea, or scream your head off. Do something that dissipates the energy you feel. Let it all out and contain the fear that you will go out of control – you won't. Don't be afraid of your anger because it is very powerful. Use it for your good. Move it into determination, resolve and purpose. Make it work for you to bring about change.

After you have done this you will feel more in control. You will feel a sense of calm and you may feel the pain that is buried beneath the anger. If you don't, then stick with identifying what angers you, because you are not sated yet. Don't worry – the pain will surface when you have made the room inside you.

Some of us possess a rage that is so fierce we are scared to touch it. If you recognise this in yourself, it would be advisable to find a professional practitioner to assist you in releasing the rage in a way that will not be harmful to you or anyone else. The section 'Get Help' (Suggestion 7) can assist you in finding someone. If you are aware that this rage sits inside you, you are halfway to taking care of yourself, as awareness takes up half of the recovery from depression.

LETTING OUT THE PAIN

Anger is usually the front end of pain. The angrier we feel, the more pain we hold. We need to let out some of the anger in order to reach the pain. Once some anger has been shifted, the pain will follow. When I have felt anger in an extreme way, it is usually associated with a sense of unfairness or hopelessness, a feeling of futility, 'how dare they', and other such emotions.

Less common is when we feel tears instead of the anger. Many people have described crying when they have felt angry, as it seemed the only way to let the anger out. These are 'hard' tears that can be turned into assertion. Those tears belong to the previous section 'Letting out the anger'. In this section we are looking at the 'soft' tears that lie beneath anger.

Again, find yourself some time and a safe place. Begin to write about what you have lost or what you have that is unwanted. Be specific and honest. Don't worry about what others might think because no one will read your words. Suspend self-judgement for the moment; it is not required. Instead of seeing yourself as a mature adult, visualise yourself as a child and write as a child would write. To further this, you may want to write with a pen held in the hand you don't usually use to write with. This helps to reach your vulnerable spot – the one that's not in control and has no limits. The sense of pain may not happen immediately, but you will be a step further towards it. This has become a lifelong assignment for me, as it helps me to reach the parts that nothing else can.

Allow yourself the gift of expressing your sadness. It won't go away by ignoring it; it will always stay with you until you express it. Indulge in the pain that lies behind the anger. Hold yourself tight as you let the tears out. Let go of the past. The more you let out, the more you will heal. Letting the tears out will free you from being stuck in the past. Imagine tears as the currency of healing – the more you let out, the more you will heal. Tears do not signify weakness; they signify trapped pain.

Allow yourself to mourn what you have lost. Letting out your pain will lead to a state of forgiveness of yourself and others. The more pain you release, the less frightening the feelings will become, and this will allow you to stop running from your fears.

Your sadness may dispel in hours but, for some of us who have suffered from chronic depression, it may be a long progression. What you will be delighted to discover is that it is the road home. Releasing the pain will only bring you closer to your birthright of happiness and contentment.

Don't worry if you don't reach the anger or pain immediately. Remember the attributes of denial and you will understand that your psyche will take you as far as you will go, only opening up the next layer when you are ready.

❊　❊　❊

5 TALK

Sometimes this works, sometimes it doesn't. It works when our depression renders us isolated from the world and we are able to tell someone about our isolation and depression and are supported. Talking to someone can act as a release valve for our feelings. We want to talk to someone who has some understanding of what it's like to be depressed. We need to be heard by someone who is not trying to get a word in edgeways, as this leaves us feeling more displaced than before. If we have someone to listen to us and not judge what we are saying, it gives us an emotional 'leg up'.

Talking to someone won't help if the other person is having a great life and doesn't know what it is like to feel depressed. Common responses from people I have opened up to while feeling downcast have included:

- Pull your socks up, you only have one life. Make the most of it.
- What have you got to be so miserable about? You have a roof over your head and a good job!
- Look at all you've got, don't you know how lucky you are? Look at all the starving children in the world!
- I know many people far worse off than you.
- Don't worry, it'll all turn out OK, you'll see.

Speak to someone who knows how you are feeling. This is when organised groups like 12-Step groups come into their own. By sharing your experiences – and hearing those of others – you can begin to come out of isolation. Find a way to feel safe in another's company by testing the water. Offer a little of yourself and your struggle, and see how you feel afterwards. The healing can begin when you feel accepted by another person. You don't need the whole world to accept you – just one person will do. This will help you to feel less 'mad'. We'll look at how to find this person in a later suggestion.

Be aware that you may feel uncomfortable when talking to others because this breaks our society's 'no talk' rule. Our culture advocates the 'no-talk' rule and praises the 'I'm fine' approach. This is because many of us are scared that someone may talk about their pain, which would be too uncomfortable or embarrassing for us. Many of us have grown up with the notion that having feelings is weak and pathetic. We have ignored them and, as a consequence, have become depressed. It is time to break the 'no talk' rule and start to verbalise how we feel. It's quite amazing how people respond to us when we open up. Indeed, the majority of people will say, 'I have felt like that too.'

It is important to be careful what you talk about and to whom you talk about it. For example, don't talk to a policeman about the crime you undertook in your darkest days. No matter how much you want it off your chest, he might not see it that way. Don't express your rage at the traffic warden who has just given you a ticket; you will feel worse about yourself in the end. It is also important to establish the difference between expressing your feelings and acting on your feelings. If you go to the doctor for help with depression, it is appropriate to talk about your feelings and your despair and pain to allow him to identify how he can help you. It isn't appropriate, however, to throw yourself onto him, bury your head in his lap and sob your heart out for a good half-hour.

It can be difficult finding the right person to talk to. If you find yourself talking to people and not getting any good feelings from it, this is where the section 'Get Help' (Suggestion 7) will be invaluable. Remember, you are not alone; there are many people who are in a similar position. According to the British Medical Association, at least 10% of the adult population is depressed at any one time – that amounts to around 5 million people.

Five Things To Do When Your Head Is Just Above Water

6 SORT OUT YOUR BODY

START WITH FOOD!

Food affects our mood. That's the bottom line! We all know that when we are depressed we often resort to comfort eating. It is really important to look at this issue when our heads are above water just enough for us to get a little perspective on the way we eat. There is plenty of medical advice available on what to eat and what not to eat, and it is often conflicting. We are bombarded by the message that eating the wrong foods can lead to illness and bad health. The problem is that when we feel depressed, what's in our fridge is of little importance to us. For those of us that can munch through a packet of chocolate digestives in about fifteen minutes, we also know that if there's one thing worse than feeling depressed, it's feeling sick and depressed.

However, if you are trying to climb back up out of a spiral of depression, you have to pay attention to what you put into your mouth. Certain foods can exacerbate depression. For instance, overdoing it on cheese, crisps, ice cream, chocolate, white bread, cakes, biscuits, coffee, alcohol and smoking can make you feel dreadful for at least a couple of days. So you need to attend to your menu.

It's easy to get into a cycle when you are depressed. You don't care what you put in your mouth, so you feel worse, and then care even less. But sometimes just being aware of the link between feeling awful and your eating pattern can be enough to spur you into action. As long as you have that awareness, the seed will germinate and grow in time.

Planning ahead is the key. If you want to eat healthily, you should shop accordingly. And if you prepare healthy food earlier, it will become second nature to get out that food and eat it. Include goodies and treats, but make sure the basics are included. I generally find that by following these two rules I can keep my focus on good food:

1 **Five portions of fruit and vegetables a day**
2 **Eat three meals a day and nothing in between**

We feel much better about ourselves when we eat well. Eating junk is part of the self-perpetuating abuse that we pour on ourselves when we have little self-worth. It's easier to fall into the victim mentality when we don't look after ourselves and then blame everyone else for not looking after us. Changing our food is a tiny step towards beating depression.

MY ONE BIG FOOD TIP – SOUPS! AND HOME-MADE IS BEST.

A GREAT RECIPE WHICH IS SIMPLE AND QUICK IS:

Soften 1 onion and two sticks of celery in a pan with some olive oil. Add 1 tin tomatoes, 1 tablespoon tomato puree, 2 cloves garlic, 1 tin canellini beans and a pint of stock. Simmer for 30 minutes then add herbs to taste (oregano is lovely). Add grated cheese to serve if you wish. This soup is nutritious and comforting and hits the spot every time.

DRUGS AND ALCOHOL

There is nothing about cigarettes, alcohol, class A or B drugs that are going to add to our wellbeing. We all know that but we still take them. This is normal when we are depressed because we don't have much self-value.

Weigh it up and work out which one to give up or cut down on to give yourself a better chance of recovery. If you can't do it on your own, the section on 'Get Help' will point you towards people who can help you. Overcoming an addiction can pull some people into recovery from depression. They have to clean up their medicating techniques enough so they can get nearer to tackling the source of the pain. But it's a 'chicken and egg' situation. The withdrawal from the drug can expose the depression – which may be why the drug was used in the first place – and if that is too painful then the user may return to the addiction.

However, there is a fantastic recovery rate for these problems with the help of Alcoholics Anonymous and Narcotics Anonymous. Also, if someone offers you the chance to go into a residential treatment centre, take the opportunity, because you will get all the support you need. There are some great centres both in the UK and in the US that offer the facilities you need to deal with drugs and alcohol. More information can be found in the 'Resources' section at the back of the book.

ACUPUNCTURE

If there is one alternative treatment to be recommended, it is acupuncture. Acupuncture involves the insertion of fine needles that carry out specific actions. This can stimulate the immune system, which will increase the body's ability to heal itself. When we are depressed we often feel unwell in certain areas of our body. We have aches and pains and feel physically down. These are often symptoms of depression, and acupuncture can help. Many GPs now offer acupuncture for patients with specific ailments, and it is becoming more readily available on the NHS. If you are looking privately, go to the British Acupuncture Council and get some good recommendations for practitioners in your area.

When you go for acupuncture, tell the practitioner that you are depressed and you want treatment for that as well as for your specific ailments. This will assist the practitioner in planning the best treatment for you. As far as cost goes, an acupuncture session starts at about £20. One session a month is good enough and it is really worth it. If you are depressed, you are probably spending money on something you can do without, e.g. cigarettes, chocolate, alcohol or drugs. One session of acupuncture can do more to change the way you feel than all your medications put together. For me, acupuncture significantly contributed to removing the grey, heavy concrete slab that had sat on my chest for 15 years. I am now free of it. That's the power of acupuncture.

7 **GET HELP**

The fastest route to beating depression is to get help from those who understand your feelings. Talking to others who have been through similar experiences to you will help you feel less isolated. Much depression is created by the negative effect that others have had on us; likewise, people who have a positive effect can accelerate recovery from depression.

We have a distorted perception of ourselves when we are depressed. We feel that something is wrong with us, that we are different from everyone else, that we are not normal and that we are alone. These things can be tackled with good reflection from other people. When I went to see a therapist, I said over

and over again that I thought something was wrong with me.
I said this for weeks and each time she would reply, 'There's
nothing wrong with you except your distorted thinking about
yourself.' Although it took a long time for this to sink in,
I came to believe her because she kept saying it. She never
budged. Whether or not I could have got through depression
without this information is a question I will never be able to
answer. However, I ate it up like a hungry infant and allowed
it to nourish me, even though I didn't believe it for a long time.

This is the kind of help we need: accurate information that
we can grasp and assimilate. There are thousands of places to go
for help, but I have simplified them into four categories, listed
below. If you take up two of the suggestions, a network will
appear and you will discover other resources available to you.

The stumbling block people often put in front of themselves
is 'it's not for me'. If this is your voice then here is the bench-
mark: If you can get good information about yourself from
your close circle then you need look no further. However,
if talking to your friends doesn't work, get help. We live in a
culture of the 'stiff upper lip' and you may not want to venture
out to meet strangers and pour out your problems to them.
When I first started talking to people about how depressed
I was, I felt really angry about the fact that I was even there.
I hated talking to others about myself and dismissed most of
what I heard for a couple of years. This is not unusual. Many
of us have to be crawling on our knees before we ask for help.
It is the nature of depression, because we feel so much shame
for needing help. If it hurts enough, we will either medicate
our feelings or find someone to help us.

FINDING A THERAPIST

When you begin to look for help, you must spend some time
getting the conditions right. This can be very difficult. Finding
the right therapist can be a bit of a lucky dip. You are going to

be bearing your soul to this person, and you need to know you can trust them. Obviously, client confidentiality is the bottom line, but there are other factors to consider. It can be a mistake to go for the first person you hear about. Finding the right therapist is like anything else of great importance – you need to shop around.

I know to my cost that rushing into a therapy situation without taking a view on the person, their working practices and the environment in which they work can be detrimental to the recovery process. I have opened up to people who needed more help than me! As an example, I went to one therapist who, in hindsight, actually had severe depression himself and would tell me about it during my session – an absolute no-no, as therapists should not be talking about themselves in your time! Together we wound ourselves into a web of inappropriate behaviour that resulted in him coming around for dinner and me counselling him on his day off. At the time I thought I was cool. In retrospect I lost all self-respect. And the bizarre thing about it was I was paying him £70 per hour!

Below are some sources of help placed into three categories:
1 Therapy
2 Unfacilitated groups
3 Facilitated groups

These three areas are to help you get started and to give you ideas of what to expect. They are not the absolute gospel, simply an idea of what's out there. Take a risk on at least one area, but the ideal scenario is to get help from an individual and from a group. The one-to-one feedback will encourage you to stop running away from your pain and will give you information on how you see yourself. The group will help you to see how others see you and also help you to feel less isolated – you will suddenly realise that there are others out there who know how you feel.

Taking a risk and making the first call is part of getting better. This is because we are doing something to help ourselves and going forward. It takes more strength to take that first step forward than to step backward by medicating the pain. This is our ultimate choice and we may swing from one to the other. We may go for help and seem to make good progress, then we decide we've had enough and go on a 'bender' for six weeks. This is common: nobody is perfect. We cannot recover overnight, it takes time and sometimes we can get fed up of waiting for change. However, any help goes towards a 'credit' in the recovery bank balance.

THERAPY

One-to-one therapy is the way to receive objective information about ourselves and our lives. It gives us an idea of what is normal and how far off normal we may be. Some people say the idea that there is a 'normal' in the first place leaves us prone to judging ourselves. However, there is a normal pattern of development that all humans go through. If we are depressed, then this pattern of development has been arrested. With therapy, we can go back to when we stopped growing, address any trauma, retrain ourselves and then heal. If we have a good therapist, we won't even realise we are going through this process – it just happens.

So how do we find a good therapist? It can be difficult, because the industry is not regulated and any of us could set up as a therapist tomorrow. Even if it were regulated, there is no guarantee we wouldn't fall in with a qualified person who also happened to be inept or just not right for us.

Therapy is different from analysis and psychoanalytical psychotherapy, whose practitioners are strictly monitored by their regulatory bodies. Therapy is a goal-orientated process that usually ceases after a set period. Analysis can last a lifetime, is more general, and more costly. Therapy can provide the treatment required for the emergency situation of chronic depression, whereas someone seeking analysis is likely to be approaching the concept of their 'self' from a more existential perspective.

The secret is to find help that is beneficial to us and does not hinder our recovery. I found the perfect therapist after asking for recommendations from counselling authorities, universities who held counselling courses, pastoral centres etc. When one name kept coming up, I took the chance and went to see her. She was the perfect 'leg up' to help me out of my depression.

There are three ways to approach your prospective therapist. First, go in with the idea that you are interviewing them. Secondly, take a tape in on the first session so you can listen to it later and assess the conversation objectively. If the therapist doesn't like it, then that's a warning signal. Thirdly, take in someone you trust to sit in on the assessment meeting and get them to give you their view later on. These tactics will sift out the weak therapists and give you a better chance of finding someone who can really get to grips with your issues and take you through some incredible changes. And it can take just a few sessions to really get an overview of where you are going with the therapist. The whole process in itself can leave you feeing better because it is the beginning of change.

What do we want the therapist to do for us?

There are several jobs that we require the therapist to undertake in order to get our money's worth.

We need the therapist to listen. Many of us have never had the experience of 'being heard'. By this we mean having someone listen carefully to our exact words and assimilate the essence of what we are saying, in order that they can reflect it back to us – so that we can hear our problem coming out of someone else's mouth. This allows us to listen to the problem in a way that lets us get a firmer grasp on our concerns. It also gives us an opportunity to put them right when they don't get it spot on.

Try this out with a friend in order to get an understanding of the power of true reflection. Ask someone to listen to you speak. Tell them what's on your mind in under two minutes, then ask them to repeat what you have said, and listen to your problems being retold. You will be amazed how this technique takes the heat out of a problem that had otherwise seemed insurmountable.

We need the therapist to offer an objectivity that we can't find ourselves. When swamped with a crisis or trauma it is almost impossible to take an overview of ourselves, as we often feel out of control and buried under a mass of anxiety and fear. We need to get an indication of our situation without being influenced by our own neurosis. We often need practical assistance in how we behave. An objective view can help us achieve this. We can make incorrect decisions about how we respond to people and situations when we are traumatised. A good therapist will help us find the right course of action that will leave us intact and will be for our own good. We must ask them to be objective on our behalf in order that we can move forward through the dilemma, outlining the options they can see and helping us weigh them up to a positive outcome.

We need a therapist to comfort us when we feel pain. Many of our problems stem from us running from painful feelings. By trusting a therapist we are allowing another human being to help us face those feelings. When we do arrive at the point where we can feel our feelings, we need support and encouragement to express them, because so many of us are frightened of releasing pain for fear that 'if we start, we will never stop'. While feeling pain or grief, we need to know we are not odd; we need to know we are going through a normal procedure of releasing our pain in order to move on; we need to know we are not the only person to whom this is happening. We do not require patronising while we move along this path, but we do require patience and understanding. The words that will soothe us are those of hope, that no matter what has happened to us we have the capability to survive and can actually create a great life in spite of our losses and our pain.

Why is this? This is because when we grieve for our loss, we grieve for everything we have lost, not just our current loss. The most important loss we can grieve is the loss of our dream. No matter what or whom we have lost, it is the dream of what could have been that hurts the most. Once we can allow the pain to surface, like the bursting of a dam our grief will also wash away so many smaller losses that have been tucked away and ignored. Well-managed grief can wash away our losses from years ago, allowing a backlog of pain to be released and for change to take place. This enables us to feel freer than we have ever felt. People often discuss the powerful spiritual experiences they have had after a time of mourning – a closeness with a God, a sense of peace, a contentment they have never had before, a fulfilment in the simple things in life. These experiences have filled many books and are often lost on the rest of us who are still running from the backlog of our life losses. It is vital to find a therapist who can understand the profundity of this journey and who can assist you in yours.

We need a therapist to explain to us what is 'normal'.
We need to know that there is a pattern of development that we are programmed to go through, that allows us to grow into our full potential. If this development is hindered then we become unhappy. A good therapist can help us by pointing out how far off that course we are, and can suggest ways we need to change our thinking and behaviour in order that we can retrace our steps and find our way out of the darkness.

For example, if we have suffered frustration in our career, a therapist would help us to explore what we need in order to feel fulfilled from our work, taking into account our individual circumstances. Likewise, if we suffered neglect as a child, we can learn what is 'normal' in terms of what a child needs, and find ways of catching up with ourselves by getting attention in appropriate ways to make up for what we've lost. If we do this, we will no longer seek it from others in ways that may be detrimental to us as adults.

Finally, we need a therapist who understands that we must grieve for a given amount of time and then stop.

It's easy to think that we are never going to recover from depression and the grief behind it. In continuing with our grief for longer than is necessary, we re-traumatise ourselves. Some therapists expect a person to be with them for years – something that will serve them well as they have a continuous income stream. No one, unless they are mentally ill, should need to be with a therapist for more than two years. Some people stay with their therapist for much longer if the therapist allows it, and this can become another dependence. A good therapist will know when we are ready to move on from our grief, and indeed may shove us out of the nest if it appears we are settling down for the long haul.

If you are doubtful as to whether or not your therapist can offer these basic services, consider finding someone else.

UNFACILITATED GROUPS

Unfacilitated groups are self-help groups that run without a facilitator. This means that they are a bit of a free-for-all, but there are some really good sources of help and support amongst them.

12-Step Groups

The most common of the unfacilitated groups are the 12-Step groups. The 12-Step groups were started by Bill W in the 1950s to help alcoholics stop drinking. All other 12-Step groups are loosely based on the original Alcoholics Anonymous format.

12-Step groups are run by volunteers, not professionals. People sit in a room, hear some opening readings, and listen to someone sharing their experience. Then the meeting is opened to allow others to share what is on their minds. The 12 steps have been adapted to embrace other forms of compulsive behaviour with a view to helping all kinds of people through the recovery programme. The meetings are anonymous and use first names only.

THE ADVANTAGES OF 12-STEP MEETINGS ARE:

- They are readily available, with a range of meetings in most towns
- They cover a broad range of subjects
- They are anonymous and use first names only, which ensures a feeling of safety through anonymity
- There's a nonchalance and informality about the problems they are covering and this can be helpful, as it may engender the feeling that we are not alone in our struggle
- For many, there's a feeling of 'coming home' when they hear others talking about how they feel
- The 'secrets' are out in the open and others talk about their sex addiction or cocaine usage as if it's ordinary; this helps dispel the shame
- They are not run by professionals but by 'people like us' and so there's a feeling of belonging
- They are all volunteers so there is no financial motive for anyone to be there
- People can be very supportive and will offer assistance to help others attend meetings
- They are based on donations only and are affordable to anyone

THE LIMITATIONS OF 12-STEP MEETINGS ARE:

- They are open-access groups (many British people aren't comfortable with talking openly about their problems!)
- There are no facilitators and you have to rely on the structure to create the right environment
- A lot of 'robust' opinions can be aired, with people wanting to tell you what to do, where to go and what to say – and the loudest voices often dominate

- **The anonymity is questionable in some groups; I know of a meeting that quadrupled in size in one week because word got around that a celebrity had attended**

However you feel about groups, 12-Step meetings can be a fantastic starting point for depression. Identify how you medicate your depression, or what you feel is the main cause of your depression, and go to the appropriate 12-Step meeting. There will be one you will fit into. It is said that when you have attended six meetings in a row, the denial will start to lift and you can better experience your core difficulties.

Here is a brief look at the purpose and limitations of perhaps the most typical 12-Step group, Alcoholics Anonymous:

Purpose

AA is designed for those who have a drinking problem and wish to give up. The idea is that you attend meetings where you listen to other people's stories and share your own experience of drinking. Support from other members is encouraged to enable each member to become sober. It is recommended that a new member attends 90 meetings in 90 days to become sober. The intensity of meetings can then reduce. The success rate is high compared to other methods of treatment for alcoholism.

Limitations

AA is perfect for those wishing to attend to their drinking problems, but for those wishing to then look at why they began drinking in the first place, e.g. childhood abuse issues, that's where the help stops. It's considered 'inappropriate' for AA members to discuss childhood abuse in AA meetings. It is also deemed 'wrong' to discuss strong feelings like anger, because the message is that we should ask our 'higher power' to take away these feelings rather than embracing them. The 'sponsorship' programme – which encourages members to ask a fellow member to mentor them – can be off-putting, as you might team up with a person who is not someone you want to be talking personally with.

Contact details for Alcoholics Anonymous and other 12-Step groups are in the Resources section at the end of the book.

FACILITATED GROUPS

These are groups that are run by a professional facilitator. There are thousands of them to be found in the UK. They range from groups for sexual abuse survivors, men's therapy groups, groups for recovering addicts, parenting groups, and groups that focus on recovery from various addictions such as workaholism, overspending, sexual addiction etc. Groups can be found in every area of the community. Doctors' surgeries offer groups run by nurses for giving up smoking; Christian centres offer groups for assisting a spiritual life-foundation; therapists offer groups for women who struggle in relationships. The list is a long one.

Like the search for a therapist, investigation and recommendation come high on the list when looking for a facilitated group. Having a therapist registered with an 'esteemed' organisation does not guarantee good service. Ask around, interview the facilitator before going into the group, don't pay for more than one session at a time and leave if you feel unsafe. Be aware, though, that we can feel unsafe in any group – we have to try and discern what is our own historic fear and what is bullying in the room.

If you find a group with a proficient facilitator and you feel safe enough to come out of your shell and expose some hidden parts, the compensation will be enormous. This method of self-exploration is the fastest route to becoming whole, as it brings to light parts of you that you are hiding from others. This is because you are taking the risk of allowing others to comment on a part of you that you assume is shameful. The exciting part is that others don't see it the way you do and they will give you a positive response. If they come back with shameful criticism, it is because they have struggles within themselves and it is then the facilitator's job to address that. Having opened up to this new type of dialogue, you will find it easier to risk something which you feel is even worse and, again, receive help and support on how to deal with that part of yourself in a positive sense. You will experience a sense of liberation as it dawns on you that there is no need to hide these parts of yourself from others. You will feel freer as you get the nod from the group that actually, you're OK!

❋ ❋ ❋

8 CONFRONT THE AUTHORITY

When we are depressed we feel we have no power. We feel no strength within ourselves and think it is almost impossible to find a new way of dealing with people that will help us in beating depression. One of the main reasons for this is that we have not confronted the authority in our life.

This means that we are allowing someone else to dictate our behaviour, thoughts or feelings. It means that someone is doing or saying something and we are obeying them. We are bending to their rules although we don't want to. We are compromising ourselves and our integrity, doing things and behaving in a way that is not right for us.

This 'authority' may be someone who is in your life right now, such as a spouse, friend, a work colleague, teacher or neighbour. Conversely, it may be someone from your past to whom you are still attached, such as a parent or sibling. You have become conditioned to believing that another person knows what is right for you. You may continue to play family games when you go back to your parents' house and smile as if everything is OK, even though it's not. This can lead you to thinking there's something wrong with you. You may have to press that frustration down so it won't escape and overwhelm you.

If you are feeling very depressed, put some thought into who it is that you are obeying right now. Are you listening to someone who gives you information about yourself that you believe? Is someone telling you that you can't go for your dreams? Are you telling yourself that you have no rights as a parent and therefore cannot have any personal life? Is someone telling you that because they give you money, gifts or favours that you have no right to confront them? Is someone beating you up and you believe it when they tell you that you deserve it? These and many other questions are worth asking yourself because there is an answer here.

HOW TO CONFRONT THE EXTERNAL AUTHORITY

Now that you have become aware that you are following orders, how do you confront your own misplaced obedience?

You could simply talk to a friend and receive valuable responses that might help you recognise your situation in a way that you can't see it now. However, if you feel very anxious about discussing your situation, you may need assistance from a trained professional who can help you see that your thinking is contaminated. Some reworking of the way you see your situation will help you to get a more level view and decrease your anxiety. This will then raise your confidence about dealing with the authority.

However, this doesn't have to be done face to face. Confronting an authority can be acted out in the safety of a therapist's room by allowing yourself the opportunity of saying to the therapist what you would really like to say to the authority. The very act of expressing your fury or sadness out loud will open you up to dealing with your depression and you will find yourself encountering new experiences that will add to your personal strength. The action you take with the authority as a result of talking it through may be simply to respond in a new way. One thing to remember – unless you break the law, there is no authority that can dictate to you. If you believe otherwise, you are misguided.

Once you have a clear idea of what you need to do or say to confront the authority, you could take action face-to-face, on the telephone or by writing; you could do it directly, through a legal advisor or with a mediator. Any route may be scary but it's the exciting scariness that comes before change and you can use these opportunities to your full advantage. Be aware that if you are depressed you may see tackling an authority as a backward step but it is not; it is a real catalyst for change and the first time you do it is always the hardest. If you stretch yourself you will give back to yourself the greatest gift of all – your personal power.

When we talk about confronting the authority, we are not talking about a screaming match in which we hurl abuse in between trying to make a point. No, we are talking about approaching it in a way that we would expect a favourite teacher or someone whom we admire to approach it. Imagine them making your point to another on your behalf. Think what they would say and write the words down as they would speak. How would they sit or stand? What would their face look like? What would their gestures indicate? Go through the conversation you imagine you will have and mimic such a person. Practise the conversation with someone who can listen and ask the question, 'Is this unreasonable?' You will discover that 99% of the time, what you are saying is reasonable and measured.

We tend to overestimate the power we have in another's life. We feel that confronting something or someone is going to throw the whole world into disarray. This is a normal part of the nebulousness of depression. We are afraid of being honest for fear that our feelings will overwhelm others. We labour under misconceptions. As I have opened up and told people things that I thought might kill them, they have hardly batted an eyelid – often the response has often been, 'Oh, I knew that anyway.' Depression distorts reality but as the depression lifts so our focus becomes clearer. There is nothing to do except be aware of it. Here is an exercise to help you confront the external authority:

Learning to say 'No, Thank You'

Many people get depressed when they compromise themselves and allow others to bully them into doing things they would rather not do. We give in to others because we are frightened about the consequences of saying 'No, thank you.' When we neglect our own needs we become empty and even resentful of others. The irony is that when we outline our limitations to people making demands of us, we feel much better about giving and sharing at other times. Some people I know have recovered from depression by simply learning to say 'No, thank you' when they are being asked to take on too much. It is terrifying doing this for the first time if we are not accustomed to saying no, because we get guilt feelings for standing up for ourselves. However, it is our right to make an honest assessment of our responsibilities at any time and, if we feel uncomfortable taking on more, we should let others know our limits. Here are some tips to get going:

- Stand in front of the mirror and say 'No, thank you' to yourself until you're bored
- Now stand in front of the mirror and say 'No, thank you' to yourself as the person you want to face
- Practise the conversation you need to have as you imagine it out loud with you saying 'No, thank you' at the right moment
- Practise with little things – even if you want to say yes to someone, simply say 'no' until you're used to it
- When you are ready, go to the person to whom you wish to face and just do it!

Yes, it's scary at first, but no more so than going to a party where you don't know anyone. If the thought is terrifying, then take a look at the possible outcomes of your actions. If you are petrified, then you are creating some archaic scenario from earlier in your life. As an adult, you are entitled to say 'No, thank you' to anything you don't wish to undertake if it does not feel right for you.

If you are going to confront the authority, you also have to be clear about your goal. Your goal needs to be about you and how you would like to feel. It needs to address what you need to get off your chest, how you want to change your behaviour in another's company, and how you want to lessen the negative effect that someone has on you.

A simple example of confronting an external authority:

Your goal may be to stop allowing yourself to feel humiliated when a colleague talks to you as though you were a delinquent teenager.

In this scenario you know that you react like a delinquent teenager, sticking two fingers up behind her back as she leaves the office or sinking into a ball of shame so that you hang your head for the rest of the day. So, you need to prepare yourself to approach the whole setup with a different frame of mind. Practise your preferred response in the mirror or with a friend until you get the right feeling in you. Next time the colleague comes in with the patronising look on her face, draw yourself up tall, perhaps stand up as she comes in, and respond to her in the way you would imagine a prime minister, for instance, to respond – with authority and firmness. Watch with interest the way your colleague changes. Accept the change with grace because you have forced it. Note the difference you feel as she is slightly on her back foot – she is used to dealing with you in one way but you have now changed your reaction to the way she speaks to you. She may not even be able to put her finger on what has changed, because you are saying the same words but in a different way. But you know what has changed, and you will soar with confidence at your courage in responding to her differently.

What your goal doesn't need to include are things about the other person. For example, this exercise is not about destroying that person, humiliating them or trying to get them to say or do something you want them to do. You don't need to confront your colleague by telling her that you are sick and tired of being treated like a child and that if she doesn't do something about it you are going to report her. You shouldn't start a whispering campaign or sending anonymous letters – it has been known! This is not a clean or progressive course of action.

HOW TO CONFRONT YOUR PARENTS

This is a huge topic and one that is difficult to sum up in the space available here. When I talk to people about depression, so many people return to the subject of one or both of their parents. I estimate that, of the people I have spoken to, 80% of them feel entangled with their parents and are stuck. For the purpose of simplicity, I would recommend two courses of action. You should take one or the other.

1. Confront them indirectly

If you know you are struggling with a parental relationship, but it is not possible, for whatever reason, for you to talk to them, find someone else with whom you can let out your frustrations. Most people would choose to take this route. Once you have established what your normal pattern of behaviour is in their presence, you can take measures to change it. You will begin to see how you still act as a child and issue the same demands. They follow your command and behave in the same way they did when they were responsible for you. But things have changed, and you have to take the lead to put the changes into place. It is not up to them to change the patterns until you ask them. The goal is to change your current behaviour when you are with them in the same way that you would confront any other external authority as outlined above.

Your first step is to identify what it is you need from them and then take steps to get it elsewhere. If you need to go to their house for the night, get some home cooking and your washing done, you are setting yourself up to be treated like a teenager. For the good stuff you receive from your parents, you must pay a price – and this is to stay in the old pattern. Get a washing machine or start using the launderette and learn how to cook your own nice meals! You then need less from your parents and you will be able to confront them indirectly as you would your work colleague, as outlined previously.

Your behaviour will gradually change and, although the change will startle them, they will adjust. What you want to achieve is you feeling better about yourself in their company. This does not entail them changing, this is about you changing. Bear in mind that it's rather like the family members being represented as bobbles on a nursery mobile. The balance of the mobile is delicate because if one bobble moves the rest are affected and all the bobbles on the mobile will move accordingly to keep the mobile balanced. When one person gets off, the mobile will bounce around for a while, before the mobile eventually settles down and forms a new shape. This is what happens when a family member puts some changes into place and forces a different dynamic between the members (the bobbles). New relationships will form and everyone will need to adjust.

2. Confront them directly

The second route to take is to confront your parents directly – a choice taken only by a minority of people. This is for those who are too depressed to 'play around bashing the cushions', because that does not do justice to what they suffered. This route involves huge personal risks because it is about confronting a perpetrator who still feels all-powerful. The point of the exercise is to diminish the power that person holds. It is not an exercise in trying to 'get them back for what they did to me'.

If you decide to take this route, make sure that you first seek professional support from a therapist and ask them if they think it would be a good idea, presuming that person would know the details of your family history. If a trusted therapist feels it would be beneficial to your recovery, you may like to consider the following suggestions for how to go about it. You could meet your parents on neutral ground, in a hotel, with a mediator, or, depending on the nature of your problem, at a solicitor's office. It would be respectful to let them know beforehand that there is something from your childhood that you need to bring out into the open. You may want to outline it in a letter beforehand.

You must be prepared to confront them without telling them how 'they' feel or who 'they' are. Instead, you will need to conduct the exchange from an 'I' perspective. This is the way of lessening the possibility of conflict, because if we tell another how we feel rather than how they feel, there is nothing to argue about. For example, if I say to someone, 'You're always criticising me,' their response might be, 'No, I'm not,' and then the whole question of whether or not they do is up for grabs. But if I say, 'I have never felt as if I have done the right thing in your company,' that is unarguable fact and cannot be disputed because no one else can know what we feel.

You may want to express your hurt and anger towards them, but don't act it out. Only discuss your tender feelings if you feel strong enough for any response you might get. Only go through with the exercise if you accept that you will not get them to change and they will probably deny what you are exposing. Don't do it in the hope that they will fall at your feet and beg forgiveness. Do it in the knowledge that the self-healing will come as a result of you expressing yourself, not in the response they offer.

If you receive a loving response, then that is your bonus. Don't fall into the denial of 'maybe it wasn't as bad as I thought'. Do it only if you are prepared to lose a relationship with your parents, even though your hope is to build a better one.

Two points to remember:

1 People are entitled to treat you how they want and say to you exactly what they want as long as they are not breaking the law. This is their entitlement. You, on the other hand, are allowed to respond to their words and actions in whatever way you choose as long as you are not breaking the law. This is your entitlement. As you practise this, you will come to realise that you have no control over other people's behaviour but you do have the power to change your response to others. In fact, your response is the only thing you have any control over.

2 By the same token, it is no one else's responsibility to change you. There is no point in waiting for someone to come along to make you do it. No one is there to sort out the way you approach others. It is not anyone else's fault that you aren't doing it for yourself. It is down to you to make these changes. The fast-track tool to help you make these changes is to confront your own internal authority.

HOW TO CONFRONT THE INTERNAL AUTHORITY

The internal authority consists of the polluted messages that you bombard yourself with. These messages are a hangover from earlier days and are no longer valid. They contain incorrect information and need to be challenged and updated. The only reason they have such a hold on you is because it has become a perpetual habit to listen to them. All you have to do to get rid of them is to replace them with a new message. To break a life-long habit, you simply need to be firm with yourself about this.

This is how to tackle the internal authority. Listen carefully to the 'polluted' message – you will know what it is because when you hear it you will feel ashamed. Catch it and study it. Think back to when you first heard it. Who said it to you? Think hard and you will find the answer. You will realise that you are obeying it even though it comes from someone for whom you may have no respect or love. If they were obeying you after many years, wouldn't you think it was a little strange? You are responsible for taking the correct course of action to remedy these old messages. No one is making you do what you don't want to do.

Next, write down the message on a piece of paper. Then put a line through it and write the antidote next to it. Stick it on the wall where you will see it all the time. If this is not possible because others live with you, then draw a picture or write it in code. As you read it, the new message will filter into your consciousness and you will find yourself adapting to it. All you are doing is changing a thinking habit – albeit a very ingrained one. In a few days the new message will be taking over from the old one.

SOME EXAMPLES OF ANTIDOTES:

I am stupid
I am not stupid, I passed my degree with honours

I am frightened I will go broke
Take that fear and, just for this next five minutes, let it go

I will never get my music deal
Your success as a person does not depend on a music deal

Just reading these through as you notice them stuck on the wall will remind you that you have an old habit that needs to be replaced by a new one, and what new thinking needs to be put into place to make a change. It really is that simple. I recommend you stick with replacing one old message at a time. Remember you must have a new message to replace the old one – you don't want to leave a vacuum. As you practise this, you will notice that when you get bored by the Post-it note on the wall it will mean you have registered the new message. Now it's time to move on to the next old message. You will find each note stays on the wall for a shorter time. It might start off as two weeks and you will move it to two days. Your assimilation will accelerate in the light of new experience. Don't make it any more complicated; that's as simple as it needs to be.

9 DIVIDE INTO THREE

Identifying some of the messages that gallop through our minds is the first step in 'dividing into three'. Dividing into three is about listening to the messages in our heads, the judgements on our shoulders and the feelings in our stomachs. It is about understanding that how we talk to ourselves makes us behave and feel the way we do.

This exercise entails grabbing the essence of your thoughts and feelings and evaluating it to determine which part of you is the directive and which part is the respondent. You will begin to see how you are controlled and, after some practice, you will find you have many more choices in how you respond to the world. When we are chronically depressed, we feel we have no choices and this concludes with us feeling hopeless.

Dividing into three is the best way to get in tune with yourself so that you can sense what is being said internally, how it affects you, and what the correcting course of action is. This stage can be very hard work, but when your spirit is in the ditch and you have tried everything else to make yourself feel better, you have no choice but to take the risk. It will provide you with lifelong opportunities to change your outlook and beat depression.

To begin to divide into three you have to make a distinction between the three parts of you: the Adult, the Parent and the Child.

THE ADULT

The Adult sits in your brain and is the wise part of you that can give you information about what is best for you without judgement or criticism. It has no emotions attached to it; it is purely objective. The best way to identify this part of you is to think about a scenario that is going on with someone you are not close to. Take an objective view about what you think is right for them. Have an overview of their situation and get a non-judging response together in case you are called up for your opinion. This is the 'intellect'. It is the sage, the wisdom or the higher self that you can develop to help you through times of decision. The voice will get stronger the more you listen. It is that little murmur you often ignore which is letting you know which direction to take. This voice sits in the brain rather than in the heart. It is the seat of all our knowledge. The Adult is a direct link to our Higher Power. The Adult transcends emotion and we can start to lean on the wisdom it has to offer as a beacon through our dark times. The Adult has only our good at heart and would never give any advice that would harm us or any other person. The Adult attempts to communicate with us at any given opportunity but this only comes in stillness – and when we are depressed we are reluctant to stop 'doing' or 'thinking'. The Adult strives to create a wholeness in us that will serve to bring together the fractured parts of ourselves.

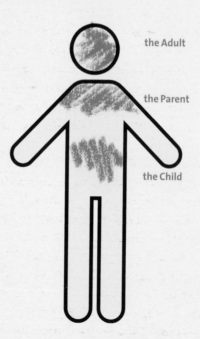

the Adult

the Parent

the Child

THE PARENT

The Parent sits on your middle torso and often on your shoulders. This is the part of you that shows judgement and can be helpful or unhelpful. You need to judge things that go on around you; you need to assess what is happening and then make conscious decisions for yourself. The Parent, like the Adult, contains no emotion, although the way it addresses you can be loving or critical. It works in a logical manner based on the map that was formed in the past.

However, the Negative Parent can often be harsh in its criticism and the severity of the criticism directly depends on how you were criticised as a child. You can hear it as the little voice in your head or on your shoulders that tells you about yourself. It will say how the world sees you and may give a regular 'See, I told you so' to reaffirm harsh condemnation that you were given in childhood. However, these messages are way out of date.

Another way of identifying the Negative Parent is to become aware of how you view others. If you think of someone you know and picture what you think of them, you are using the Parent. It is important to be aware what those thoughts are because how you view others is generally how you view yourself. You can only see the world as a reflection of yourself and it is a good guide to understanding how you are to others. You need to have this Parent inside you but you have to change it so that it becomes a softer Parent who makes assessments and guides you with a firm but gentle voice.

A man was talking to his three-year-old daughter who refused to put on her coat as they left the doctor's. He bent down and talked to her at her level. He then said, 'We have to put on your coat because it's very cold outside; now shall we do this firmly or gently?' After a whole minute, during which the man just sat, the little girl said, 'Gently' and held out her arms. This is the touch we need to give to ourselves. We took on the script that our parents fed us whether we wanted to or not. As children, we had no choice. But as adults we can change the way we talk to ourselves because we now have the power to do this.

The first step is just to recognise this 'Parent'. Whether it is a loving voice or a horrible voice, for the moment, don't try to change it. This voice is your 'ruler' for better or worse. It is the voice that judges you – for good or bad. This voice is the intermediary between your 'Adult' and your 'Child'. It is not always rational – indeed it may never be rational. It is a mirror of your parents' authority. This may be to your good, but if you have become very depressed then the chances are this parental voice needs some adjustment.

We need the Parent inside us to become a good judge. We need to make judgements on the world to protect us. People who have well-developed judges trust themselves when dealing with others. They are relaxed in others' company because they don't feel threatened. This is how we have to develop the Parent in us – to become a good judge of ourselves and others.

THE CHILD

The Child is your feelings or emotions. This is the part of you that cries, laughs, feels joy, anger, frustration, jealousy, rage and pain. Your Child will live in your torso, which extends from your ribcage to the bottom of your stomach. Different parts of your torso may hold different feelings. Fear often lives in the top of the stomach or in the ribcage; joy often lives in the bottom of your stomach.

The state your Child is in is dependent on the relationship between the Adult and Parent. If you are depressed it's because your Child has had no voice or good Parenting for some time, maybe never. Many chronically depressed people encompass a traumatised Child. This is a Child who has had to withhold the possibility of joy because it feels dangerous to need love or want contact with others. Children who have been neglected or abused will not trust adults; similarly, our own Child will not trust our own Adult for care and guidance, and we respond to the world like a child who has been let loose.

Conversely, if we begin to develop our Parent self, using the methods I have outlined, we will better access our Adult self to give us the wisdom we need to take care of ourselves. Our Child self will feel less isolated and will trust a little more. Learning to talk to ourselves is the fastest route towards building self-trust and, although it is difficult in the beginning, we must persevere. Once we have learned to do this, we have a skill that will keep us moving forwards toward our higher goal.

✳ ✳ ✳

10 LEARN TO TALK TO YOURSELF

Learning to talk to yourself is the basis on which you can move yourself forward and away from your depressive state. Talk to yourself through the Adult, Parent and Child. Once you begin this practice you will easily identify the different parts of yourself, and you will pinpoint the voices that are creating your depression.

To illustrate the power of talking to yourself, take a moment out and relax. Recognise something that is a big worry in your life. Think about the worry and recognise the negative feeling that you have in your Child part. Sit with this feeling for a moment. Next, from your Adult part, find the antidote that would make your worries go away. Now, imagine that the antidote has been put into place. Really, really believe that it has happened and whatever was worrying you isn't there any more. Now feel the difference in your Child.

This shows how powerful thoughts can be in that they can dominate us. The exciting discovery is that you can change the thoughts that affect the way you feel. It really is this simple. You have the power within you to succeed whether you believe it or not. The difficult part is breaking old habits that have been with you for a long time. The habits are often lifelong. But they can be changed.

Examples

Some examples of problems and antidotes follow. It may help
to write yours down:

Problem: I am afraid that people are judging me when I get to the
school gates.

Antidote: That thought stems from way back when you were a child and
you felt judged every day. That may have happened then but it is not
happening now; in fact you have no evidence that people are judging
you. You are imagining a scenario that is completely outdated and it is
time to look at the actuality. They are probably more concerned with
judging themselves and what others think of them. When has anyone
ever made it clear that they are judging you? Having said that, if
someone does judge you, it says more about their insecurity in your
company than it says about you. It's time to brush that thought away.

Problem: I am scared of losing my home and living in a cardboard box.

Antidote: I understand that you feel that way but that thinking is the
power of your invention. No matter how tight things have been
financially, between us we have always found the resources to ensure
our home and bills have been paid for. You have had that fear for about
twenty years and at no point has it ever come true. You are
scaremongering and we have to put that thought away because there
is no evidence to support your belief.

Problem: I will never feel anything but hopeless.

Antidote: I can feel the hopelessness in you and I appreciate that it is
very depressing. However, you have felt this way before and it has
passed. You have come away from feeling hopeless and, let's look at the
evidence, you have actually touched on joy. It feels more familiar for you
to stay feeling hopeless because it's been with you, on and off, since you
can remember. But this is not your natural state and you will move away
from it again. Just be patient and, remember, this too will pass.

You can now start to see the Child part of you as an actual child because, emotionally, this is how you really are. Many of us still react to the world in a childlike manner, especially if we are depressed. To understand this, imagine yourself today with a small child by your side. Every time you need to respond or deal with someone, this child is responding on your behalf. If you are depressed, this part of you will not be equipped to deal with the world in an adult way. If you appear as an adult to others, it is common to feel like a fraud.

The maturity and happiness of your Child is paramount to beating your depression. Take some time out to imagine this part of you. How old is your Child? Is she happy or sad? Is she afraid or confident? What is she wearing? What facade is she presenting? Ask yourself these questions and you will gain great insight to your soul. Once you have begun to get a glimpse of this Child, you can start to mobilise the Adult and Parent to help her grow up.

If we are depressed it is because we are stuck. We need to learn to re-parent ourselves with trust, humour and love. This is why we may seek other people's help – we are not sure what is 'normal'. When we go for therapy, we are paying for a 'Parent' to teach us how to re-parent ourselves. This is why it is so important to find a good therapist in order that you do not damage yourself further.

Get into the habit of talking to yourself as you would like to have been talked to as a child. If it becomes the guiding tool that you turn to when you are depressed, then you will gradually stop the downward spiral of depression.

If you have been depressed for a long time – in my experience more than two years – you might find this exercise difficult, because the Child in you does not trust the Parent in you.

A simple exercise to start this process is to look back over the last year and identify what you feared would go wrong at the start of the year. Write these fears on a piece of paper. Then, identify what actually did go wrong and write this down as well. You will find two things. One, your worst fears didn't come true, and two, what did go wrong was unexpected. Your trust in your judgement was misplaced. People often do this. We focus on what *may* go wrong. We become anxious about something that *may* happen. It is an easy habit to get into. This is where we need to employ our reason by removing the thoughts that generate fear. Most of our fear is based on something that *might* happen.

This approach to learning to trust ourselves is no different to the way we would strive to build trust with an abandoned child brought to our home for us to look after. We would see a frightened child who trusted no one. We would have to work hard to build a relationship that was based on firmness, fairness, love and consistency. Over time the child would open up in the knowledge that she could take steps towards you, ask for what she needed and expect to receive much of what was asked for. As the child's confidence grew, she would become softer, gentler and more fulfilled. She would become more playful and excited about life. She would return the love and respect tenfold. This is our payoff. This is how we will feel if we talk to our self as a wounded child.

We may need to show our Child evidence that we are up to the job. As the trust grows, we will recognise the opening up of our soulful self and the quest for contentment will be underway. As your Child becomes more trusting and confident in the world, you will experience a joy that comes with confronting a real or imagined authority. You will open parts of your spirit that you didn't know existed. You will enjoy the company of others without needing to compete. You will discover the secret of happiness is found simply in being alive.

Tackling Shame

Tackling our shame is at the crux of our recovery because shame is the root of self-loathing. When we feel stuck and imprisoned, it is shame that binds us to our depression. When we experience shame we are not open to the world, we cannot receive from others, we don't trust ourselves not to fall apart if we talk about it, and we feel of little value.

Shaming is something that we experience as children. If we feel deep shame we have a hangover from the way an adult has habitually addressed us in a cruel way. Adults are constantly shaming children. You see it everywhere. Just walk into any supermarket and you can see a child being called some foul obscenity or suffering some awful humiliation. As adults we continue to talk to ourselves in this manner. If we hadn't been shamed as children, we would not take it up as an adult. It just wouldn't happen.

SOME EXAMPLES OF WHEN WE MIGHT FEEL SHAME ARE:

- Too often we feel we are doing the wrong thing at the wrong time, e.g. we turn up at a party wearing full evening dress when everyone else is in jeans
- We expose our weakness, e.g. when someone sees us cry
- We feel less than we are, e.g. we simply don't feel good enough in others' company no matter how many times they tell us we are great
- We judge ourselves harshly, e.g. at the school gates, a works 'do' or our local gym, when everyone else looks as though they have the perfect life and we feel like a social leper
- We feel we have been exposed, e.g. we accidentally send a bitchy email about someone to the person we were vilifying when it was meant to go to our best mate
- We feel we are living a lie and we must do everything and anything to keep up the lie to the point of exhaustion

When we feel shame we believe that the very core of us is contaminated and needs to be kept a secret because, if it gets out, it may contaminate everyone else. Shame grabs our head and pulls it down so that others can't see us. Shame leaves us believing that we are worse than anyone else. Fear of being found out about how shameful we are drives our lives. All our actions are governed by how we can dodge being 'found out'. Being 'found out' means the end of us because we couldn't survive the humiliation.

When our shame becomes unbearable our denial will kick in. This will render us incapable of feeling the shame. But this may become a temporary life-saver (although it may not be others' preferred remedy for helping us) until we feel better and we can face reality a little at a time.

However, until the shame is confronted we are trapped. This is because, as children, we could not confront our persecutors because we needed them for our very survival. The shame that was bestowed on us is still in charge. But as adults we have choices and we can heal this shame.

The healing must start from a different place to healing other parts of our trauma, e.g. our grief. Healing our grief starts when we feel backed up against the wall with nowhere else to go and we feel forced to confront our pain. Healing our shame comes from the opposite corner because we need to feel a little safety and security before we can possibly open up to our shame. The very nature of shame is its ability to hide at the drop of a hat with denial, quickly setting us up to say, 'There's nothing wrong with me!' or 'This is not happening,' or 'I have no idea what you're talking about.'

HEALING THE SHAME

The key to healing our shame is to expose it. Shame is like a bacteria that needs to be kept in the dark to grow. Opening ourselves up and letting in some light will kill off some of the shame. Shame left in the dark multiplies.

Start by exposing it to yourself. The following exercise will help you uncover your shame, allowing it to come out of its hiding place. You can then begin to tackle it by addressing it with your Adult self. Look at the table and its examples below. Draw an outline of the table in your journal and follow through the instructions if you feel ashamed about something. Don't worry what others might think – it is not intended for anyone else to read.

The exercise contains a suggestion that you open your shame to another person ('Expose it to another'). Only do this if you have someone, or a group, who will listen without judgement. If you have not found that place, wait until you find it.

What am I ashamed of? Let my Child do the talking	Expose to myself why I feel like this	Employ my Adult self to expose the truth	Expose it to another	Take action by employing my parent
I feel ashamed because I boasted to my friends	Because I felt inadequate in their company and I wanted to feel superior to make myself feel better	I am not inadequate and I do not need to boast about my achievements to prove this	I will explain how I feel and how I use boasting in a number of occasions to boost my self-worth	When I next feel like boasting I will tell myself I don't need to put myself above others to feel OK; I am an adequate person the way I am
I feel ashamed because I pretend I have more than I do	Because I think no one will like me unless I have wealth	Being wealthy does not bring friendships. In fact it can keep people away from you and maybe this is what you need at the moment	I will open up to my feelings of loneliness and share the emptiness that I fill up with self-pretence	I will begin to grieve the absence of accepting myself just the way I am; I will work towards self-fulfilment by comforting my sad and lonely Child

Healing shame involves getting to the heart of the pain. You will find pain you didn't know you had. In the first example in the table, the pain of needing to boast comes from the anguish of feeling worthless without the prop. This is painful because, like a child, we cling to a fantasy that we have to 'do' and 'own' to be accepted by others. We believe that no one will like us if they know what we are like inside. But with accurate counselling from our Adult self we can come to terms with the pain and view it in a new light. We can see that this is a childlike reaction to the world that keeps us from the world and from our potential joy.

As you begin to expose things that you feel ashamed about, you will feel better about yourself and will find yourself wanting to expose all of it. It's as though you have cleared out a messy drawer that you have been avoiding for years. Now you want to get the rest of the drawers cleared and then tackle under the bed. The feeling that comes with exposing shame is liberation.

LOOKING AT OUR BEHAVIOUR

Another way to tackle shame is to look at our behaviour and identify how it has both protected and enhanced us. The goal is to take steps towards bringing the lighter side of our behaviour more into focus and thereby diminishing the way it has created negative patterns.

In this exercise you have a grid with four columns. You must identify your behaviour pattern, how it has had a nega-tive influence, how it has protected you and, finally, how it has enhanced you. Don't judge yourself – that's not important. What is important is that you can identify your behaviour, because our depressive behaviour has both negative and positive aspects to it. We have behaved in ways that have protected us and it is time to learn how we can alter our behaviour to our best advantage. That is the ultimate responsibility that we can take for ourselves and it will engender compassion and reduce anxiety. Some simple examples are outlined below:

My Behaviour	The Negative Influence	How It Has Protected Me	How It Has Enhanced Me
I am messy	It keeps my brain fuzzy and unable to gain clarity	It keeps me feeling calm and keeps me busy so I don't need to address my problems	It has taken me away from depression by giving me another fixation
I am always angry	I have lost the trust of those close to me. I have been out of control	It keeps me from getting close to others and therefore my own loneliness	It has enabled me to express my frustration and let it out rather than eating me up inside
I am aloof	I have lost my own sense of self by pretending things are different to the way they are	I can feel better than others, which has given me temporary relief from my own shame	It has kept me from closeness to others which I have not been ready to bear
I say when I am depressed	I have driven others away who could not handle my depression	It has kept me from having to feel 'happy' when I'm just not up to it	It opens me up to my real feelings and helps me move forward towards security
I am kind and considerate	I have ignored my own needs	I haven't had to expose my own needs – which has felt unsafe	I have received good feelings through others' gratitude

When you begin to outline your modes of behaviour, you will start to feel respect for yourself. You will begin to see that your behaviour has worked well for you in many ways by keeping you safe from the outside world. You will begin to recognise that you can expand on the positive traits of your behaviour while reducing the negative ones. For example, although being messy has helped you to stay busy, you can start to take steps to clear up some of your messiness, which will bring you some peace of mind. If you are always doing things for others, it may be time to stop unnecessary good deeds and concentrate on performing more good deeds for yourself. Your negative traits may have been learned as a child and served their purpose well. If you are recovering from depression, then the negative behaviour has outstayed its welcome and it is time to say good-bye. You have new tools to change your behaviour patterns and the self-destructiveness. Your negative behaviour will diminish as you appreciate how to turn your actions into positive enhancements. This will heal the shame that goes alongside the negative behaviour.

❊　❊　❊

Dealing With Children When Depressed

This subject is a hidden topic. It's the one we don't discuss because we don't have to – it all takes place behind closed doors. Abusive parenting can happen when we get depressed. The madness of depression is that it happens even though we would give everything for it not to happen. In the depths of the suffering, we lose some self-control and are likely to affect our children in ways we regret. Untreated, depression will drive us towards treating our children in the same way we were treated. Abuse doesn't just mean physical or mental violation; it also means neglecting, taking no interest, not disciplining, not listening, not loving or simply not being present. Take a moment to read the 'Bill of Rights' at the end of this chapter and absorb the words. Not only do you need to fulfil your rights in adulthood, you also need to fulfil your children's rights in childhood.

KAREN'S STORY

Karen's 15-year-old son is, on the outside, a tribute to her. He seems happy, gets good marks, is in the top set at school, has friends and enjoys his sport. People often say what a lovely boy he is. Karen adores him and is concerned that her depression in his early years has left its scars. When he was a toddler, she was desperate and would scream at him to watch the television and not get up until it was finished because she needed some time to herself. She was short-tempered and intolerant of him being so little and helpless. She admits she was violent in her demeanour towards him – although she never hit him. It was her hardness towards him that fills her with so much concern. She now has so much more peace within herself that, in hindsight, she can see her intolerance.

She had never talked about it with anyone but, during an honest conversation we had about our children, she opened up as never before. Her son rarely talks about his feelings and is always 'fine'; he is competitive to a frightening degree; he is so ashamed of failing that Karen worries he may harm himself if he doesn't reach his standard of perfection. He is also extremely aggressive towards her. It may be the natural behaviour of a 15-year-old, but there is a legacy of mistrust and low self-worth in the teenager.

On the other hand, Karen has minimised the damage of her depression as best she can and, at the end of the day, sometimes we have to accept that this is as far as we can go. As painful as it is, we have to acknowledge a degree of power-lessness over passing on our legacy. The way we treat our children is the most harrowing subject for us to talk about, but we are not alone and there are more and more resources to help us to look after our children when we are at rock bottom.

Here are four suggestions for parenting your child that I learned from a child specialist while going through just this anguish. They helped me grasp some simple notions that I was able to manage while feeling like I was drowning:

15 Minutes per Day

Children need full-time care but, as far as attention goes, they need at least 15 minutes of undivided attention a day. This 15 minutes needs to be spent with the adult's focus on the child and on nothing else. It needs to be spent doing something the child wants to do. During this time, the child needs to feel respected and cared for and the adult needs to suspend all negative feelings about the child. The child needs to feel that whatever she says or does, the love shown to her is unconditional and unquestioned. She needs to be the focal point of the adult's enjoyment for that time. Something as simple as doing a jigsaw with a toddler or sharing a cup of tea with a teenager will get the conditions right to carry out this commitment. It doesn't have to be much. Even though this seems like an obvious thing to do, when we add up the time we spend with our children, many of us are not spending 15 minutes of unadulterated time per day with our children, depressed or not. This is our gift to them.

If you cannot spend that time with your child, they are being neglected. Find someone else to do it. This could be a family friend, neighbour, childcare specialist or your partner. Explain what you want the adult to do. The adult does not need to love the child but can demonstrate a clear respect for the child as a unique human being in their own right. Get the conditions right for the carer and allow the adult and your child to share the time together. You can be there and watch and know that your child is getting what they need.

Once your child begins to receive that 15 minutes a day, they will become more 'full up'. As their worth increases as a result of receiving the undivided attention, they will be less draining on you. In turn, you will find looking after them easier.

Trust Them

Children know what they need and they will make their needs clear. We have to trust them. If they need exercise, they will badger us to go out. If they need food they will ask until they get some. If they are tired they will let us know. If we ignore their needs, we get badly behaved children. We must also trust them in terms of their own limits. They know they don't want to go down the big slide yet; they don't want to be pushed into the pool even though they've got armbands and a rubber ring on. Respect their limits and trust they know what's best for them. If we don't, we are pushing them for our own requirements not theirs.

It Is Not Personal

It is the job of a child to push whenever they can. This is how they learn – through experimentation. There is no other way to learn what is acceptable and what isn't. They have to accidentally spill the milk to discover that it is better to keep the cup away from the edge of the table. However, when we are depressed, we can see the spilt milk as a personal threat and respond accordingly. As teenagers, they may express their embarrassment at being seen with us and we could take this as a personal affront, especially if we are also an embarrassment to ourselves.

But it is not personal. Whoever their parents turned out to be, they would go through the same motions. It is their way of pushing the limits and it is our job to teach them how far they can go. We must be aware: how we approach our children is the way we approach ourselves.

Good Discipline

Children like to be disciplined. They like to know where the edge is. It makes them feel safe because they can stretch to that point. They can see the boundary of the field and they are not scared of running to the edge and looking out. Children who do not receive good discipline are frightened. They don't understand how far they can go and they become anxious that they will get punished for something when they didn't know the limit. This creates fear and a lack of confidence. The limits need to be spelled out, written down, discussed and shown over and over again until they are bored of hearing it. This will create a haven of fairness, trust, safety and reliability that will allow them to grow into confident children. Many towns now have parenting groups, which can be very helpful.

CHILDREN'S BILL OF RIGHTS

This is a list of basic human needs that I believe every child has a right to:

- **To be fed (with nourishing food) and watered**
- **To be safe, warm, sheltered and secure**
- **To be touched, held and caressed**
- **To be loved unconditionally**
- **To be respected as a unique human being, regardless of behaviour**
- **To make mistakes**
- **To ask for what they need**
- **To say they don't understand**
- **To change their minds**
- **To decline responsibility for another's problems**
- **To express their feelings**
- **To be happy**

❊   ❊   ❊

The Question Of God

I want to briefly address the question of a God and how our beliefs may play a part in our overall wellbeing. We can develop a great sense of consolation from the belief in a God or some other form of spirit greater than ourselves. This has been borne out since time began and needs no further justification. However, if we don't believe in a God, there is a different way to approach the question of a Higher Power.

It is worthwhile allowing the Child in us to believe in a God if it feels emotionally valuable to us. Children love the idea of a God, or believing in some greater power. This may be an angel, the nature of the universe, fate or a spirit guide; it may be the Adult wisdom inside our self. Accepting such a notion could remove an area of anxiety (such as, 'What's going to happen to us if we can't pay the rent next week?') that can be dealt with in due course. In the meantime, the belief can provide a comforting ambience, which can help us when we are in so much need of reassurance.

It is possible to incorporate two principles into your belief system. There is a God for the benefit of your Child but there is no God for the benefit of your intellect. You can develop your position for your own best advantage. Some people have had such a traumatic time that any belief they may have had has been smashed, so trying to develop their God is destructive. Others may have never even considered the notion and may start from scratch. Whatever your stance, cultivating a belief that there is something out there which is more powerful than yourself can liberate the Child from believing that humans are all-powerful. Children don't want to feel all-powerful because it is unsafe and too scary.

When you are distressed, talk to your Child self and soothe yourself by reassuring her that there is a greater being at work. This will offer your Child an instant sense of relief and bring back into focus the fact that you cannot control anyone else, only yourself.

We need to learn to relax in the belief that everything will turn out OK. We can relax, even if the world around us is in turmoil, because ultimately all things pass and there is more to universal creation than human drama. We all go through crises; we make mistakes we think will never be rectified; we lose people, money and possessions, and these experiences can feel devastating but, ultimately and universally, everything will still turn out 'OK'. When we are stricken by grief and suffering, we can find some respite by considering a more esoteric, spiritual worldview that does not place the human individual at the centre of the universe. If we can shift our consciousness a little to the point where we are not so immersed in our own personal circumstances, we can expand our awareness and find comfort from a Higher Power or Universal Law. Practising this thinking can enable us to feel calmer in times of trouble. We will come to the point where we accept turmoil as challenge and exploit it for our own opportunity for growth. Nothing will be insurmountable. We can learn to tell ourselves, 'It's all just stuff,' whether we are going through the highs or the lows.

When we feel powerless, we can think back to a time when we sat with similar feelings and note how we came through it. We begin to mobilise our reason and sense and employ it to talk to our Child self in the knowledge that our worst fears are only imagined. We have previously used our Adult self to reason our way through fearful times. We know that it is our Child's fear and lack of trust that drives away any idea of a faith that things will be OK. We have to teach our Child self that there is a bigger picture to our life. We can show our Child the evidence.

If we are depressed, we don't have much trust in our Adult self. This is because the Child part of us has, for a long time, been allowed to run wild. This cycle has to stop and this is achieved by finding the wise voice within us to contain the Child's fears. Even a thread of an idea that things could be OK will be enough to start the ball rolling. When we are depressed we find this the hardest notion to accept. But we must work hard to find the starting point and push hard to perpetuate it.

Once we have taken the first step towards reasoning on the side of there being a more powerful being than our childlike self, our faith in things turning out for the better will grow. As time goes on, we will find that we are naturally talking to ourselves as a wise sage and actually letting go of our fears, knowing that they are simply fears and not reality.

Some of the happiest people I know believe that there is an all-powerful being to which they surrender their lives but, at the same time, they are pragmatic. They stay focused on their day, unwilling to worry about tomorrow because their Child self is trusting and happy in the wisdom that it will all turn out right in the end. Their secret? Plan but don't project.

✳ ✳ ✳

One Amazing Thing

There is one amazing thing you can do that will change the way you feel within hours. When you feel depressed, close your eyes so that you can see the Child in you. If you have trouble getting that vision, then get a photograph of yourself as a child. As you see your Child, pay attention to your feelings. They may be turbulent and vigorous.

Go to your Child and, if she will allow you to, pick her up. Take her into your arms and soothe her with the voice of your loving Parent. Become a therapist to the Child by imagining what a therapist would say to the Child. Talk her out of whatever is troubling her. Tell her that everything is going to be OK. Explain that she is reacting to something that is imaginary and that no harm is going to come to her. Find the antidote to her anxiety and give practical examples of how her worst fear is unfounded. Use your Adult reasoning to bring this information to her. Take as long as you need until your feelings change.

This is all you have to do to feel immediate results. With practice you will find yourself doing this exercise regularly. You will feel some comfort usually within minutes. If you are consistent, you will find comfort on a regular basis.

We are speaking to the core of ourselves. This is the way we can work through our depression from the inside out. If we post notes around our house to remind ourselves to do this whenever we need to, we will remember to do it more often. If we live with others and would be embarrassed by this exercise, then we write something in code, draw a picture or put it only where we can see it. The more often we do this, the better we will feel. We will become increasingly proficient at this technique until we are doing it on the bus, in the car and eventually when we are conversing with others. It will help us to respond more to the world as an Adult and less as a threatened Child. We can restore confidence to ourselves and we will learn how to reconcile things that worry us.

It is a little piece of magic and people who do this live in a state of joy. They rarely allow 'stuff' to affect them. They don't get depressed and they don't live their life through others' values. They live life in a state of feeling powerful, without wishing to abuse others, in control and full of fun. They have great respect for themselves and, in turn, they have great respect for everyone else. This is how we reclaim our life.

❊ ❊ ❊

The 12 Promises

Recovery will happen in hindsight. There will be no firework display that lets us know we are home. There will be no band playing for us as we walk into our house one day. As recovery takes place, we will only see it as we look back over time and realise what has changed. We will see how we behave differently in a familiar situation. We will look back and laugh at things that used to paralyse us. We will be amazed we ever felt like that. We will wonder at our previous dilemmas and feel pride in the way we handle them now. We may feel the tears when we remember the desperation that we used to feel. We will be able to put our finger on two or three specific moments that got us started on the whole journey. We will feel such gratitude that we had the strength to get to this point. We will thank the 'whatever there is out there' that helped us through the dark times.

Here are the twelve promises adapted from 'Adult Children of Alcoholics & Dysfunctional Families' that will come true if we follow the ten suggestions to beating depression and reclaiming our lives:

1 We will discover our real identities by loving and accepting ourselves

2 Our self-esteem will increase as we give ourselves approval on a daily basis

3 Fear of authority figures and the need to 'people-please' will leave us

4 Our ability to share intimacy will grow inside us

5 As we face our abandonment issues, we will be attracted by strengths and become more tolerant of weaknesses

6 We will enjoy feeling stable, peaceful, and financially secure

7 We will learn how to play and have fun in our lives

8 We will choose to love people who can love and be responsible for themselves

9 Healthy boundaries and limits will become easier for us to set

10 The fears of failure and success will leave us, as we intuitively make healthier choices

11 With help from the support we have put into place, we will slowly release our destructive behaviour

12 Gradually, with our Higher Power's help, we learn to expect the best and get it

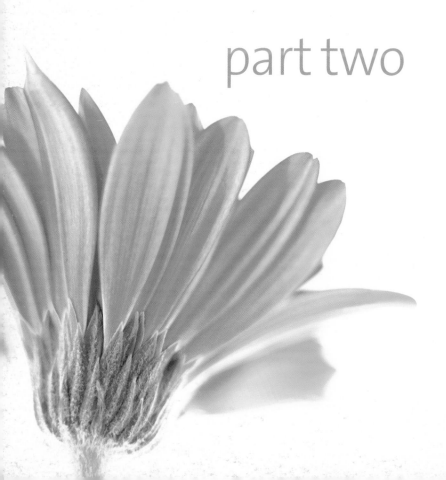

part two

The 14-Day Plan to Beat Depression

'When a person acts without knowledge of what he thinks, feels, needs or wants, he does not yet have the option of choosing to act differently.'

CLARK MOUSTAKAS, HUMANIST PSYCHOLOGIST

Sometimes we need another person to tell us where to go, what to do and what to say. We can become confused and disorientated when we suffer from depression. There is no obvious route to recovery. If we contract a major illness, for example, cancer, we are aware that there is a medical route for treatment and we probably know that there are various complementary therapies that are approved by the medical profession to help alongside traditional treatment. But if we are depressed it is hard to know where to go to receive help. There is little publicity about treating depression and the very nature of this state of mind renders us unable to think clearly, become assertive and demand assistance. When all we want to do is curl up in a ball and hide, it is very hard to force a sense of clarity out of ourselves.

This is a plan to help you find that clarity and meaning in your current state of mind and offer ways to sharpen your focus on moving out of depression. Whether you simply feel low or you are negotiating a way out of years of depression, this 14-day plan is adaptable to you. Each day offers tasks that will help you to feel better. You can move on to the following day when you feel you have had enough of the previous day's tasks. Conversely, you can jump ahead and try something that shines out at you.

If you are simply feeling a little low, you may want to skip through the 14 days in as many hours. If you undertake the tasks, you will find you feel more confident, your depression will have lifted and you will have a bounce in your step. If you have suffered from depression for a number of years, you may want to take each day's tasks on for some weeks at a time. Stay with each task until you feel saturated and you have had enough. You will be moving yourself in the right direction rather than floundering in a hopeless vacuum. If you decide to follow the plan through in 14 days, just like a 14-day diet, at the end of it you may not have lost all your 'weight' but you will have the tools you need to get to your goal.

The whole of the 14 days is designed as a sequence of tasks that can help to lift you up to the next step. They are written as a way to place the Ten Suggestions from Part 1 in a manageable order that will create a sense of moving forward. They are designed to encompass everything you need to recover from depression. There are hundreds of other tasks you can undertake, but these 14 days take in the fundamental path that you must follow to completely recover from depression.

PREPARATION

The Journal

Before you start you will need to get yourself a journal. This will be your workbook, and it will hold the answers you are looking for. Don't use a scrappy old notebook or something that looks as if it was designed for an accountant. Get hold of a nicely designed, sumptuous book that gives you a lovely feeling when you open it. You can fill your journal with personal treasures: the beautiful leaf you came across when you found the energy to go for a walk; a particular fragment of material or a design that caught your eye; things that are aesthetically pleasing to your psyche. It will also contain your writings and thoughts and will be the document that charts your recovery. Treasure it.

Time Off

Before you start, look at taking time out. Reduce your responsibilities. Book yourself two weeks of not doing very much. Take a deep breath and bite the bullet. We all deserve a break and, if you are reading this, then it's probably your turn.

If you flounder at this point because you can't reduce your responsibilities, take a look at why not. We are not created to be a slave to other adults; our responsibilities are towards our children and ourselves. If you are depressed and have too much responsibility to take time out for yourself, this may be why you are depressed in the first place. It would be a good time to challenge your overall level of responsibility.

Goals

Before you begin your 14-day plan, it is a good opportunity to state your goals, or what you would like to achieve by the end of it.

Open your journal and write down the scenario in which you would like to see yourself. Paint a picture of your dream life. What would have to happen for your life to get back on track? Maybe you were never on track and this will be your goal. Maybe it will be living on your own or simply liking yourself. Maybe someone you know who is sick will get better, or that your own health will improve.

Whatever your scenario, write it down. We all know deep in our hearts what needs to be achieved to help us move forward and reclaim our life. This will be the first item in your journal. It will be the first thing you see when you open your book. Make sure it's really what you want and then write it down.

DAY 1
Take The Day Off

However deep or light our depression is, a day off is good for all of us. Even if we think that this applies to everyone else but us, take a day off anyway. Beating our depression can simply be about putting ourselves first. Some of us can turn the corner by this one, simple objective and a day off can help us achieve this.

What are we taking a day off from?

We need to take one day off from our duties. This means we need to go out and play. It doesn't mean we take a day off work and then clean the house or do the odd jobs that we are desperate to get finished. It means we do something that used to fill us with joy and we haven't done in a long time. We must be self-indulgent and do one big thing for ourselves. Here are some examples:

- Go to a park
- Take a long, warm bath with candles and scents
- Have a massage
- Go on an early morning hot-air balloon flight
- Go on a picnic
- Visit the seaside
- Walk in the country
- Paint a picture
- Book a ride on horseback
- Write to your heart's content
- Sleep all day
- Climb a large oak tree
- Take a dog for a long walk

We find it very hard to do these sort of things when we are depressed. We think we don't deserve it, we haven't worked hard enough, or we simply don't have the energy – in which case we can simply lie down for the day.

SURRENDER

When you learn to fly a plane, you have to become skilled at managing the controls: the rudder, the elevator, the throttle and so on. It can become quite a tricky business making sure all the controls run as they are meant to. If these controls are not operated in symmetry, the plane and the pilot can enter a flat spin from which only a very experienced pilot can climb out. Once the plane is in that lethal situation, it takes real skill to recover from it.

A Cessna, however, is a common plane in which to learn to fly. If you get into difficulty, or a spin, and you don't know how to recover from it, you simply let go of the controls. This gives the plane the opportunity to sort itself out because it is designed to be dynamically stable. When learning to pilot a Cessna, the instructor will get you into a muddle and then ask you to let go of all the controls. Naturally, it is easy to feel a sense of fear as you do this, but then a sense of calm takes over as the plane adjusts to being free of unnecessary interference.

This is how we surrender – we let go of control. We are running from our painful feelings and sending ourselves into a flat spin. Just let go and allow your spirit to re-balance itself.

Deep inside us, no matter how hidden, we have a stable spirit. We are designed to move forward, grow, develop and mature. It is part of human nature to love, experience loss, grieve and accept. It is the gift of life that we can experience bliss and joy.

However, we are inclined to interfere with this natural cycle by trying to control how we feel, ignoring our emotions or using something to suppress our pain. We do this because we are sure the depression will catch us up and devour us. But it won't – it will simply keep us on the run. Once you hold your hands up in surrender, you may feel overwhelmed by the strength of anguish that follows. Do not despair; this is a backlog of sensations that have been building up.

Thoughts of suicide

Some of us are frightened that if we surrender then we may
not survive. These words are for you.

In our most depressed state of being we can experience
thoughts of suicide. We may feel ravaged by the world and
think that the only way out is to stop living. Surrendering to
our depression in this state may seem like a foolish thing to do.
But running from these thoughts may harm us more because
it is the running that wears us down. We become too foggy-
headed to make clear judgements.

Thoughts of suicide can hit us for two main reasons: either
the pain is too much for us to bear or we are so enraged with
other people that we want to punish them. In either case we
have given up trying to protect ourselves because we have
failed in the past. We feel backed into a corner and there seems
no other alternative. All reason has gone and we are at a loss to
see any other option but to take our life and end the suffering.

It is at this point that we don't want anyone else to try to talk us
out of the way we feel. When we have suicidal thoughts, people
may say things like this:

- 'Oh, come on, it's not that bad'
- 'Don't be silly, you don't really want to do that'
- 'Pull yourself together, you're talking like an idiot'

When we hear those kinds of comments we want to show them
exactly what we mean. It can fuel the desire to commit suicide
even more and become very, very unhelpful.

If you have thoughts of suicide, surrender to the feelings
that lay behind the thoughts. A technique to help you do this
is to look down to the floor. This will help you to 'feel' whereas
looking upward helps you to 'think'.

Behind your thoughts lies the utmost pain that any human
has to bear. You might feel the intensity of human degradation,
the devastating pain of loss or the wretchedness of a lifetime's

neglect. You might feel your spirit has dried up and your essence has been ripped away. You might feel like a 'nothing' or a 'very bad person'. You might sense that everything you touch, you damage. You will probably be living in a dark tunnel. You might hate every part of you as much as you hate others. You might feel a desire to injure others as you have been injured. You might want to destroy others as you have been destroyed. You might simply be lost.

Whatever the passion is, then just for today stay with the feelings and ignore the thoughts or the action.

Just for today hold yourself around the tummy as you recognise the emotions behind the thinking.

In this moment acknowledge that you feel so bad that you want to end your life. Don't do anything else except surrender into it. Tomorrow you can take action, but just for today, surrender. Hold your hands up and give in to the feelings. Say out loud, 'I surrender'.

At the lowest point of his depression, Michael felt as though he couldn't continue because the pain of life was too hard to bear. He took an opportunity to speak to someone he trusted, Scott, and this is the essence of what he said:

> 'Michael, I understand that the pain is so great that you want to take your life. I can see and hear that you are considering this option. I recognise that you see this is the only option for you.
>
> 'If you die, I will come to your funeral. I will grieve for the man for whom I had so much compassion and respect. I will be devastated but I will also respect that this was your choice and your right. I will tell your daughter what a wonderful father you were and how you always tried your utmost. I will speak in your honour and I will talk of our friendship without betraying you. I will keep your trust and honour your memory. You will be greatly missed.'

This was what Michael needed. It was the fact that another human being was able to see and recognise that he was in so much pain that he was considering leaving his life and his child because he could hardly tolerate it any more. Scott didn't try to talk him out of it but accepted his thoughts of suicide. This was Michael's 'levelling out' – he had hit the bottom. He was then able to tell himself that, yes, it was that bad. From that moment, he was able to surrender to the emotions and allow the pain to rush through him like a rocket. This is the essence of surrendering. It is about paying tribute to ourselves. It is about saying, 'I have had enough; I can't tolerate any more.'

Some of us can reach inside ourselves and some of us need others to help us reach inside. Only you will know what your need is. People I have spoken to have stated that they felt so suicidal that they abdicated responsibility for themselves in order that they would become 'medically sectioned'. This is more common than we realise and is a route that some people take if they feel unable to move beyond this point.

Some of us don't come through it. Sadie couldn't surrender to her depression and, after a long period of isolation, she committed suicide at home having organised her friend to come around that afternoon and find her in the bath rather than one of her two children. She left devastation behind her. That was Sadie's intention and it was fulfilled.

This is the reality of depression. A few of us don't survive. But most of us do. However, we want more than simply to survive. We want fulfilment and fun, love and excitement, fairness and simplicity. This is our right and this is what we are striving to achieve. We can survive thoughts of suicide and come through them. Thoughts of suicide do not mean we will commit suicide; it means we are asking ourselves to stop and listen. It is the thought that we are at the end of the trail, and it is time to listen to ourselves and ask others to listen to us.

What Might Happen When We Surrender?

When we surrender to our depression, we may experience strong feelings that we didn't know were there. We should not despair. These are feelings that we have been running away from. We don't have to summon our courage to face them because if we are at this point, then we are already able and willing to face them. We have reached a point where we want to move forward and so our denial will have shifted enough to address the feelings that are lying in wait to come out.

The overwhelming feeling that arises when we surrender is 'Thank God!' This is because we have faced the truth that all is not well inside us but we are no longer willing to lie to ourselves. We might feel immediate relief and respite as the weight of holding the dam wall together dissipates. We can tell ourselves that we are actually OK; it is simply that we are depressed. While this phase takes place, we must do whatever it takes to see ourselves through these first days. We can take ourselves to a safe place and relish the freedom from anxiety as the weight of denial lifts.

How long should you surrender for?

Undertake this first exercise until you feel some new energy entering you. You may have been depressed for months, in which case you may feel one day is enough. You may have been depressed for many years and need to undertake surrendering for much longer. Take up to a week and incorporate a sense of surrender every day. Put by an hour a day to contemplate what you have been going through. Do this while reading a gentle book, taking a warming bath, meditating or lighting a fire. Find something soothing to do while you contemplate your thoughts. Don't judge yourself – there are good reasons for how tortured you have felt or still feel. You will come to feel ready for the next step as you gain acceptance of your pain and fear.

DAY 2
Surrender

Make this your first task today. Surrender to the powerlessness.
Be aware of the hopelessness.

Today, acknowledge that life is difficult. We tend to think
that everyone has a great time except us – this is the isolation
that comes with depression. But in reality, many people find
life to be a difficult and arduous journey. Once we begin to
accept that life is difficult it feels less difficult. We might hide
our depression when we hear comments such as 'What's
wrong with you?' 'Why aren't you at work?' 'What have you
got to be depressed about?' This makes us feel under pressure
to appear OK when we feel dreadful; and when we get home,
we feel worse. Much depression is brought about by high
expectations and, in accepting that life is difficult, we can
readdress some of that pressure.

WRITE IT OUT

'The great thing to be recorded is the state
of your own mind; and you should write down
everything that you remember, for you cannot
judge at first what is good or bad; and write
immediately while the impression is fresh,
for it will not be the same a week afterwards.'

SAMUEL JOHNSON, 1773

It is important to get some time to yourself to tackle the start of your writing. It is necessary to harpoon the essence of our depression and translate it into words, and we therefore need that focus. We must press ourselves to settle and concentrate on ourselves, harness our energy and begin the education of teaching ourselves to beat depression, starting with our journal.

Take out your journal and open a blank page. Be aware that this journal is going to contain many secrets – you will need to find a safe place in which to keep it so that you will feel free to write all you want into it. As you look at the blank page you can be sure that this is the start of change. Write this heading: 'Why Am I Depressed?'

Begin by writing down exactly what it is you're depressed about. We generally know what we are depressed about and, surprisingly, we can usually fit it all into one paragraph. Sum it up in your own words.

Once you have completed this first part, you may want to ponder the answer and debate your situation. Read your paragraph again and you will see it as a confined problem. But we know that the power depression has to emanate from us and surround us in a way that makes us feel utterly powerless. How can a problem that can be summed up in one paragraph create so much havoc and destruction in our lives?

Now you must answer some questions. Don't concern yourself with why you need to answer these questions – simply surrender to the process laid out in front of you. Write out each question in your journal and answer it fully. This task may take you half an hour or it may take you weeks. It makes no difference on the timescale, only that you answer the following questions:

- **Who/what is holding me back?**
- **Why are they/ is this holding me back? (write three examples)**
- **What is it they are doing to me? (write three examples)**
- **What effect is this having on me?**

Again, give thought to your answers and be clear and concise as you write. A picture will start to emerge as to your status quo. You will begin to see some objectivity within your feeling of helplessness. You will find a common thread that runs through the answers. We will address these answers another time. Today, think through the reasons but don't act on them. The more honest you can be with yourself, the more you will gain.

❋ ❋ ❋

DAY 3
Surrender

Today, surrender to the utter powerlessness you feel. Just for today, surrender to the futility of all your efforts to remove the depression from your life. Today, just give in and give up. It is not a weakness, indeed, it is a strength to admit that we are overpowered. Surrender to your inability to run from your depression any more.

WRITE A JOURNAL ENTRY

From this day through to the end of your recovery, undertake at least 15 minutes of writing every day. This is best carried out during an undisturbed period when you are alone and safe.

Write about how you are that day. Don't judge yourself but write it as it is, no matter how awful it seems or looks. Try writing with the hand you don't usually use. This acts as a powerful stimulus and can trigger thoughts we didn't know we had. It also takes time to write with the other hand, and we therefore tend to get to the point more swiftly.

The therapy is in the writing, not the reading it afterwards. Sit for 15 minutes a day to undertake the writing, even if you only manage one line.

There are some exercises in the next 11 days that require writing in the journal. These exercises are over and above the 15 minutes a day. These are meant to be remedial, constructive and to enlighten us about ourselves. They are not compulsory and are meant to be undertaken only if they will produce some good information to help us move forward.

CRY

'Grief itself is a medicine' WILLIAM COWPER, 1782

As we begin to surrender to our depression and write about it, the denial – which we have needed to protect ourselves – may start to come loose. The denial has been keeping us safe by protecting us from our painful feelings. Added to this, the running we have done to keep ourselves away from our pain is lessening as we surrender to the depression. As a result of surrendering and writing about our depression, buried memories and feelings will surface. This may seem alien to us; we are not used to staring our feelings full in the face and we may get scared.

Crying lessens pain
Pain that is stuck keeps us depressed, but crying helps shift this stuck pain. The strength comes in releasing our pain. But because we are used to burying pain rather than letting it out, it has clogged us up. The more we release our pain, the more we are released from depression. The greater we cry, the greater the release. This release will filter through to us within 24 hours of a cry. This is the art of good stress management.

What do we cry about?

When we are depressed, we can easily feel that we don't have
what we really want, that others have what we want and that
life's not fair to us. We may not have our own house, children,
good health, a partner, money to spend, the right job, etc. If
we yearn and pine for what we haven't got, we set ourselves up
to fail our own expectations. We become angry with ourselves
and others for not getting what we want. In turn, the anger
will settle in us and render us depressed.

The fastest route out of this cycle is to cry for what we don't
have. Behind that grating resentment is pain. Behind every
seemingly impossible situation when our backs are against the
world, we have lost something. When faced with these losses –
over which we have no control – we can either stay angry,
confused and helpless or acknowledge our loss (or perceived
loss) and let out the tears.

When we let out the tears, we can make the most of that
moment by thinking hard about everything that we have lost
that has felt so precious to us. Surrender to all the clinging-on
hopes that it 'might change one day' and let the sadness of the
fact that you don't have what you want wash through you.
Experience the dawning that you may never have it and feel
the slump in your spirit that you may have been living a fantasy
to think that it was ever coming your way. Don't judge yourself.

It is easier, but more damaging, not to face this pain, and
our society dismisses the idea of shedding tears as a way of
growing up. This is why so many of us are depressed and
down at heel in spite of everything we have.

The pain that feels most familiar to those of us who have
suffered from a long depression is the pain of never really
having the childhood we yearned for. It is the pain of feeling
utterly alone and abandoned. It's the misery of experiencing
life's deep disappointment. As a little child, we hoped and
prayed that things would change and get better, but they
may not have. It is the pain of isolation that we felt at being

completely let down. This pain is the deepest we will ever feel and sits closer to our soul than any other. But if we allow ourselves to feel it, it is also the fastest route to recovery from depression.

How do we know when we have reached that pain?

We know when we have reached the pain from which we are running because it feels like there is nowhere else to go. We know that we have reached it because it is as deep in our bodies as possible.

How long do we cry for?

Cry for as long as it takes. Some people need a couple of days to cry; others may take longer. This depends on the length of the depression that we have suffered.

However, we never cry as much as we think we will cry. It is surprising how little of that deep, searing pain from which the tears of healing spring we need to feel in order to beat depression. Having asked many people the question, 'How long did you cry for?' I have put together some examples of how long others needed to cry to heal certain parts of their depression.

What needed healing	How much crying it took	Over how long
The loss of the father we never knew	1 hour per day	4 days
The break-up of a 7-year marriage	Collectively – 2 hours per week	Six months
Sending a child to boarding school	Maximum of 1 hour per day	1 week
Loss of a partner	2 hours per day lessening to a minute per day	2 years
Losing a beloved pet	3 hours per day lessening to 10 minutes from time to time	Over 1 month

When we are stuck and we think we will never recover from a loss, it is often because we find it so hard to confront that searing pain. We find that when we do reach it, we stay there for only moments at a time. We feel so good afterwards that we may wish to stay there for longer in order that we cleanse ourselves totally. We have to be patient and pace ourselves. As long as we surrender and lessen our methods of medicating our feelings, our natural development will take care of this powerful healing process.

What if I can't cry?

If you cannot reach your tears, do not fret; your psyche is not ready. If you want to reach your tears and you can't, your anger will be covering them up. Anger and pain are like the ends of a seesaw. When one lies low, the other swings high, but they both live in us, and they directly affect each other. For the moment, concentrate on expressing your anger and frustration; the pain will come. There are ways to encourage this process.

Firstly, find a photograph of yourself when you felt vulnerable and study it. Cast your mind back to when the photograph was taken and remember how you felt. Feelings don't leave us and our mind can always recall those times. Give it to someone else with whom you feel safe and ask them to describe how they see you in that photograph. There is nothing like gentle reflection from someone whose comments we appreciate to offer a picture of ourselves that we can't always see.

Secondly, write about something you have lost and read it aloud to someone who matters. If you haven't got access to anyone, then record your story on a tape and play it back. As you listen, feel the emotions in the bottom of your stomach. Practise these two techniques and this will help you to release deep pain.

If we think about our lives, we spend most of our waking hours trying to do everything we can to avoid facing our emotions. From the moment we get up to the moment we drift off to sleep we are on the move – doing, doing, doing. That's without actually medicating our feelings with work, shopping, sugar, alcohol etc. It is more likely that we aren't in touch with our feelings than that we are able to access them at will. So, don't fret if you feel numb for sometime. Your feelings will surface as you slow down, surrender and write it out.

Having beaten depression, I now find that it only comes back when I eat badly. That's bottom-line stuff to remember! The next section deals with diet and hopefully will inspire you to really make a difference to the way you feel – with instant results!

Surrender

Why do we continue to surrender and what is it exactly we hope to achieve by surrendering?

We easily lose sight of life's simplicity. We can move into a compulsive mode where we need more and more stimulus to take us away from our pain. Then we feel lousy for mistreating ourselves and this adds to our misery.

Surrendering to our depression is about putting our hands up and waving the white flag at the enemy – our racing mind. It's a way of saying 'Stop – let me out, I've had enough!' It's about colliding into the padded crash barrier and staying there, not bothering to get up. It's about getting off the racing track and admitting you've had sufficient hairpin bends for a while. We can bow out of the race with dignity because we have other things to do.

The normal human path of development that helps us grow up and mature concentrates on us shedding old baggage in order to move forward. Just as a snake must shed its skin in order to progress and survive, we constantly need to shed old habits, longings, yearnings and ideals for us to mature and experience the true gift of life – life itself. As we shed old ways, new ones fill the space and these new dimensions bring us peace, fulfilment and joy.

WRITE A JOURNAL ENTRY

Write an entry into your journal about what you are surrendering today. Write about your racing mind and how it constantly competes, rendering you confused and exhausted. Make a list of all the things you are trying to control, for example, your weight, your husband's drinking, your wife's infidelity, your next promotion, etc.

Now give all these things an importance rating from 1 to 10, from 10 for a 'life and death' issue to 1 for a trivial matter. List them again in order and draw a line between numbers 5 and 6.

All the things at 5 and below you can drop. It doesn't matter what they are, it's time to drop some areas of your life that you are trying to control. You cannot move forward until you have more mental legroom to help yourself. To let go of these things, you have to find a replacement way of behaving. Next to the bottom 5 areas we are trying to control, note down how you are going to behave when you are tempted to take control again. For example, trying to control your children's school grades: your new behaviour may be to help with homework, if asked, and give loads of praise for good work or reports. If trying to control your weight, your new behaviour is – just for today – eat three meals a day and nothing in between, together with 5 portions of fruit and vegetables, and STOP thinking about losing weight.

We have to stick these reminders all around us because our habit to try and control everything is so strong that we will never remember to replace our controlling urges with new behaviour unless the reminder is right in front of us. Write your replacement behaviour on your wall, on a note in your briefcase/bag/pocket, on your screensaver (coded if necessary) – anywhere so that you can't get away from the fact that you need to change.

The startling thing is that it doesn't take that long for change to seep in. Within 48 hours you'll notice that you are behaving differently and your approach to the bottom 5 is a little more mellow. This will reduce your anxiety. As you become more proficient at this exercise, move up the list, one by one. You'll find it less necessary to control other people, places and things.

Sort Out Your Body

The beat depression food plan for nourishment and wellness

'We live in an age when pizza gets to your home before the police.' JEFF ARDER

We all know that alcohol 'slows you down' while coffee 'picks you up'. Despite all the evidence suggesting that good food can provide huge benefits to our emotional wellbeing, we continue to eat foods that offer a short-term comfort but inject a longer-term setback. I once ate a large tin of Quality Street when I felt too depressed to move. That night I felt drugged and the next morning I felt worse than ever. I knew I would feel like that yet I ate them anyway. Which is insanity. This section is one of the most important in the book – what you put into your body will really affect how you feel. This is the time to take control and instantly help yourself to feel better. There are some foods that are well known for their ability to affect our mood, our levels of alertness, anxiety and stress, and the chemical composition in our brain. This is said to be because the nutrients in food are precursors to neurotransmitters – the chemical messengers that carry information from one nerve cell to another like, 'I am anxious'. Added to this, foods are made up of more than one nutrient. How different nutrients interact will define the production and release of neurotransmitters.

Despite this complexity, we can roughly divide foods into those that most affect depression and those that can support recovery. Foods that most affect depression include sugar, wheat, caffeine, alcohol, chocolate and dairy products. Foods that most support our recovery from depression include water, vegetables, fruit, oil-rich fish, whole grains, fibre and protein.

There is established knowledge of how food affects us and they are as follows:

- Protein can boost alertness and can give us a slight mental boost. High protein foods include fish, poultry, meat, eggs, green vegetables, cheese, milk and tofu.
- Carbohydrates can help relax us and create an anti-stress effect. Research has shown that dieters tend to become depressed about two weeks into a diet due to a decreased carbohydrate intake. Eating carbohydrates will trigger the release of insulin into the bloodstream, which produces a sense of calm and, after eating a large quantity, induces sleep. Carbohydrates are found in whole-grain bread, rice, pasta, crackers, cereal and fruits.
- Caffeine – evidence has shown that one or two cups of coffee a day can add a lift and is an unusual stimulant in that it does not require more doses, day by day, to get the same effect. Any more than two cups a day can be counterproductive.
- Folic acid deficiencies have been linked to depression in clinical studies. Psychiatric patients were found to have a much lower level of folic acid than the general population. Just 200 micrograms was enough to relieve the symptoms of depression, which is obtainable from a portion of cooked spinach or a glass of orange juice.
- Selenium. A lack of selenium has been shown to cause bad moods and causes anxiety, hostility, irritability and depression. The right amount can help us feel better and, to get a daily dose, we need one brazil nut, a tuna sandwich, a handful of sunflower seeds or an avocado pear.

It's all very well hearing the facts but, when we are depressed, we couldn't care less! But at the same time, we do want to minimise our self-abuse. My personal experience has also been that when I overload my digestive system with junk food, I feel bloated, sluggish and more depressed. And when I eat a good diet, I feel lighter, more energetic and cleansed. But we are bombarded with so many 'good eating' plans that it is hard to get serious about one. This is well documented within the slimming industry, which is continually being criticised for perpetuating the yoyo effect among slimmers – the 'losing weight, gaining weight' syndrome. We become fatigued by the facts that are thrown at us, and each new one becomes a little less eye-catching. The easiest way to organise our diet is to concentrate on health.

REMEMBER: FIVE PORTIONS OF FRUIT AND VEGETABLES A DAY

If we simply adhere to this rule, we find ourselves feeling better – not only because of what we are putting in our mouths but also for what we leave out in order to fit in the fruit and vegetables.

WHAT TO DO FIRST

The first thing to do is not to dread change. Any change that takes place can be as slow as we want and as gentle as we want. In order to get our diet to include the FIVE rule, we need to plan ahead. This is the key because, when we don't plan, we have nothing to eat and we dive for the junk and end up feeling worse.

Plan your menu for 3 days at a time. Ensure your meals include the FIVE rule. Then shop for it. Here is a 3-day menu plan to follow:

BREAKFAST

It is said that breakfast is the most important meal of the day. It lines the stomach and gives us the energy we need until lunchtime. Our preferences for breakfast differ, so below are four suggestions to choose from:

1   Whole porridge oats simmered with soya/rice/goat's milk or water. Mix in some sultanas, prunes or nuts. If required, sweeten to taste with maple syrup or honey.

2   Sugar-free muesli. There are some superb mueslis available in supermarkets that are sugar-free and have a minimum wheat content but are high in nuts and natural fruit. Eat them with dairy-free milk.

3   Fresh smoothie. If you haven't already got one, invest in a hand-held blender (the best gadget invented for the kitchen) and make up some gorgeous smoothies for breakfast. You can find packets of 'summer fruit' in the freezer compartments of supermarkets. A handful of these fruits are convenient and quick for smoothies and they also chill the drink. Some recipes are as follows:

MANGO & SUMMER FRUIT: Place 1 chopped mango and a handful of 'summer fruit', topped with juice or non-dairy milk, into a blender and mix together until smooth.

BANANA & PRUNES: Place 1 banana and half a tin of prunes in unsweetened juice into your blender. Add fruit juice or non-dairy milk and then blend until smooth.

4   Fresh fruit salad. Make up a fresh fruit salad to last 3 days. It's so easy to dive into a plate of fruit first thing in the morning if it is already made up.

FRESH FRUIT SALAD: Chop up 1 mango, 2 kiwi fruit and 2 apples. Add a handful of seedless grapes, a tin of pineapple chunks in unsweetened juice, a tin of prunes in unsweetened juice and a handful of strawberries.

LUNCH

The most delicious and warming lunch is a bowl of home-
made soup or stew. This can be made in advance and then
frozen in portions, taken to work in a flask or dipped into
when hungry. The great thing about making a large pot of
soup or stew is that it is available to us when we can't be bothered to cook for ourselves, particularly when we feel low and
depressed. Make up two pots of soup and stew every week
and freeze some of it into portions so you will have a variety
to choose from. Below are recipes for Minestrone Soup,
Leek & Potato Soup and Bean & Vegetable Stew.

THREE RECIPES

MINESTRONE SOUP

2 diced carrots

2 medium onions, finely sliced

1 finely chopped stick of celery

100g of smoked ham/bacon
(optional)

Olive oil

Oregano

2 finely chopped leeks

2 chopped potatoes

1 can plum tomatoes in juice

2 chopped courgettes

350g chopped French beans
(2cm pieces)

1.5 litres fresh stock (or 2 stock
cubes in 1.5 litres water)

1 can haricot beans or chickpeas
in unsalted water

A handful of small pasta shapes
or broken spaghetti

Parsley

Percorino cheese (the sheep
equivalent of parmesan)

Sauté the carrots, onions, celery and ham (if using) in 5 tablespoons
of olive oil until glazed. Add 1 tablespoon of chopped fresh oregano
or 1 teaspoon of dried oregano. Add the leeks and potatoes. Stir until
coated with oil. Add the tomatoes, courgettes, French beans and stock.
Cover and simmer for an hour and a half. Add the haricot beans or chickpeas
together with a handful of small pasta shapes or broken spaghetti. Simmer
for another 15 minutes. Add parsley to taste and serve with percorino
cheese (the sheep equivalent of parmesan). Makes 8 portions.

LEEK & POTATO SOUP

3 medium leeks	1 litre vegetable stock (fresh or a cube)
2 medium potatoes	Small bunch of parsley (chopped)
1 medium carrot	Olive oil

Wash and chop the vegetables. Heat the olive oil in a thick-bottomed pan. Add the carrots and coat with the oil, then add the potatoes and allow them to sweat with the carrots for 5 minutes. Add the leeks and sauté for another 5 minutes.

Add the stock and simmer for 15 minutes with the lid on. Turn off the heat. Add the parsley. Put the lid back on and allow the parsley to wilt for another few minutes.

Take off the heat and blend with a hand blender until smooth. Season to taste. Serves 4 large portions.

BEAN & VEGETABLE STEW

4 tablespoons olive oil	400g sweet potatoes
2 onions, chopped	3 tablespoons paprika
2 carrots, chopped	2 teaspoons cayenne pepper
2 teaspoons caraway seeds	1 small can of tomato purée
4 peppers, chopped	1 litre stock (fresh or cube)
350g French beans, topped, tailed and cut into 2cm pieces	2 cans borlotti beans, drained

Sauté the onions, carrots and caraway seeds in the olive oil for 5 minutes. Add the peppers, sweet potato, paprika and cayenne and sweat them together for another 5 minutes. Add the stock, tomato purée, French beans and borlotti beans and simmer for a further 30 minutes. Season to taste. Makes 8 portions.

If you just cannot find the time to make soups or stews, some of the supermarket brands are a good substitute. The ready-made salads are also great for a fast-food lunch and beat the stodgy, cardboard experience that a sandwich gives you. But when you prepare one of these dishes at home, or open your flask at lunchtime and savour your meal, you will feel the comfort of home cooking seep into you and nurture you. You will feel satisfied and virtuous! And you will remove the craving for sweet or stodgy food.

SUPPER

We tend to look forward to supper, as it's the time of day when we are most relaxed. However, nutritionists stress that eating a heavy meal in the evening is not good for us. Going to bed on a heavy stomach can give us a restless night, as the digestive system works overtime to absorb the food. Below are three sample recipes that are easy and light, with the added advantage of being dairy-free and wheat-free.

THREE RECIPES

ROASTED VEGETABLES

This dish is very filling and leaves you with that satisfied feeling of having had a full meal but knowing it's done you good at the same time.

In a roasting pan, place:
4 chopped carrots
3 chopped parsnips
4 quartered, medium red onions
10 button mushrooms
2 sweet potatoes
6 quartered tomatoes
2 cloves of garlic, crushed

Add 1 tablespoon of your favourite fresh herbs (thyme works well), or 1 teaspoon of your favourite dried herbs. Dribble 2 tablespoons of olive oil onto the vegetables and coat them with your hands. Place into a hot oven (200°C) for 45 minutes.

5 minutes before the end of the cooking time, crumble 100g of goat's cheese and put back into the oven, allowing it to brown. Serve on its own or with a salad. Makes 4 portions.

SALAD NIÇOISE

125g sliced runner beans

10 small new potatoes

4 hard-boiled free-range eggs, shelled

300g tuna steak

1 small bunch of basil or your favourite herb

1 bunch of salad leaf e.g. lamb's lettuce, sorrel

12 halved cherry tomatoes

1 small, finely sliced red onion

5 anchovy fillets

the juice of 2 lemons

olive oil

seasoning

Simmer the new potatoes until soft. Drain and halve them. Slice the runner beans, place into boiling water for 2 minutes then plunge straight into cold water to stop them from cooking any further. Divide the tuna into 4 pieces and place in a hot pan coated with a little olive oil. Cook until you have reached the right texture: 1 minute for rare, 2 minutes for medium and 3 minutes for well done.

To serve the salad, first divide the salad leaf between 4 plates then add the potatoes, runner beans, tomatoes, anchovies, onion and olives. Place the tuna steaks on top of each pile of salad. Cut the eggs in four and place them next to the salad. Mix the lemon juice with the olive oil to taste, season and drizzle over the salad. This can be served with rye bread, some other wheat-free bread, or on its own. Serves 4.

SWEET POTATO CURRY WITH CHICKEN AND BEANS

This is a simple but delicious curry dish that will appeal to the whole family. If the chicken is not wanted, simply replace it with a packet of baby sweetcorn.

300g sweet potatoes, peeled and cut into small chunks

2 tablespoons olive oil

1 onion, finely sliced

4 chicken breasts
Small jar of Patak's Balti Curry Paste (283g)
300g pack French beans, halved
250g cherry tomatoes
1 small pack fresh coriander

Heat the olive oil in a large, thick-bottomed pan and fry the onions until lightly browned. Cut the chicken into chunks and add this to the onions. Seal the meat for about 2 minutes.

Stir in the curry paste, thoroughly coating the chicken. Add 600ml hot water from the kettle and reduce the heat. Allow to simmer for about 10 minutes with the lid on. Add the sweet potatoes and simmer for 5 minutes. Add the green beans and simmer for a further 10 minutes.

Season to taste. Just before serving, add the cherry tomatoes and coriander and allow to infuse for 2 minutes. Serve with steamed rice and chapattis. This dish tastes even better the following day. It can be put in a flask for lunch or frozen into portions. Makes 4 servings.

SNACKS

We all need something to munch on when we feel down. But it's easy to reach for things that will make us feel worse rather than better, like chocolate, sweet biscuits, cakes, cheese, etc. Because these foods can have the effect of medicating our feelings, we trick ourselves into thinking we will feel better but we don't, we feel worse. Here are some good alternatives for snacks:

- **Fresh fruit**
- **Fresh vegetables (e.g. peeled carrots, radishes)**
- **Rice biscuits**
- **Oat biscuits**
- **Raisins or sultanas**
- **Plain nuts**
- **Packets of unroasted, mixed fruit and nuts**
- **Toasted sunflower seeds**
- **Dried apricots, prunes, pineapple etc.**

Put these snacks in lovely jars in the cupboard. They will seem appealing and yummy to look at, which will put us off diving for the cooking chocolate in a bad moment.

Rule: Three Meals a Day and Nothing in Between

Many of us have found that sticking to this general rule has helped us get a grip on our eating habits. If we start by getting our meals in place, we will find that much of the chaos that follows those of us who neglect our eating habits will calm down. When I started applying this rule, I felt as though I was doing something wrong by eating three whole meals a day. But, having got a handle on that, I discovered that I felt good when I ate regularly and I felt even better when I incorporated 5 portions of fruit and vegetables a day.

The plan starts with breakfast. In today's world, the pressure to be very slim is bringing us more stress than ever, and skipping breakfast seems like a good way to cut calories. But skipping breakfast is also a way of neglecting ourselves. By 11.30 we feel lousy and need a stimulant to pick us up, and so the cycle begins. No one escapes this because our bodies all work in the same way. You won't be immune to mid-morning hunger just because you are fashion-conscious.

For some of us, eating breakfast seems naughty or indulgent. We are used to ignoring what we need and it can take a long time to allow ourselves to eat well. But getting a good breakfast down us is one way to get the whole day's eating plan in place. If we mobilise ourselves to do this along with planning for three days ahead, we will see some remarkable changes in the way we feel. After a while of good and consistent eating we start to see some of the following happen:

- **We generally feel more balanced**
- **We feel less depressed**
- **We have more energy**
- **We crave less junk food**

- We sleep better
- We feel less stressed and anxious
- Panic attacks decrease
- We recognise the benefits of good eating which motivates us to continue
- We feel much cleaner inside and this has a profound effect on our emotional state
- We gradually feel our bodies change for the better

Dealing with cravings

When we are depressed, we crave things to medicate our feelings. In our darkest hour some of us can only reach for the chocolate, fat or sugar. But we can begin to plan a menu when our head is above water and we have just enough energy to see to the next three days.

The 'three meals a day with nothing in between' rule (including 5 portions of fruit and vegetables) will provide us with less cravings. What we then do is halve the amount of junk food we ate yesterday. In doing this we will feel even better on day two and we can halve again the amount of junk food we had the day before. Even if we maintain this for only three days, we will have the experience of feeling healthier and more vibrant. We can carry on the three-day plan in our own time and by our own choice.

This method of eating is easily incorporated into our day once we get started, and doesn't tie us down to a rigid arrangement that we can't adhere to, where we may find ourselves tripping up at the first hurdle.

In time we will come to relish the 'cleanness' we feel inside and we will see weighty fats and large amounts of sugar as unpalatable. We will have more energy and we might need to find more activities to absorb this extra energy.

EXERCISE

Exercise is the most effective way of physically changing how we feel, and it requires the most amount of effort. When we exercise, endorphins are released into the body and this boosts the mind and spirit.

'Exercise' is a huge subject and is personal to each individual. We need to give our heart a work-out to produce the 'feel good' endorphins that will occur as a result. If you are doing no exercise at the moment, then a fast walk three times a week may be what you need to feel better. However, if you are already fit, then a game of squash or an exercise class three times a week may be what you need. Many leisure centres now have well-equipped, reasonably priced gyms with qualified staff to help plan an exercise routine for you. If you're worried about how much exercise to start with, consult a doctor or a personal trainer.

Yoga

If you aren't keen on the idea of jumping around in a gym, then yoga can be the perfect answer to getting a total mind/body outing without having to sweat for it. It is calming, non-competitive and gentle. It is also perfect for relieving the symptoms of stress. Even the smallest towns have a yoga class somewhere as part of the local adult education programme. There are many forms of yoga being taught these days, brought to prominence by celebrity endorsement, but the basic Hatha yoga is the one to aim for if you have never tried it before.

After a period of time, usually a couple of weeks, the benefit of exercise for those who are unused to it can be astonishing. Not only do the right chemicals get released, but stamina and strength increase. In turn, we carry ourselves a little taller, we feel fitter and our mood will lift.

Exercise may be just what you need to help you absorb the extra energy you will feel from changing your eating plan. However, if you find you only have the energy for one or the other, just take each task a day at a time.

ACUPUNCTURE

I have already mentioned acupunctue in the first part of the book, but it is worth mentioning again. A survey conducted by The Daily Telegraph found that scientists in fields ranging from molecular biology to neuroscience were twice as likely to use complementary medicine than the general public. Three quarters of scientific users believed they were effective, with acupuncture topping the list. The method of acupuncture – seems strange to us in the Western world, but it is really worth checking out. Personally I have found acupuncture to have an 'unblocking' effect, both physically and emotionally. I simply feel as if everything is flowing more freely.

There are ways to receive acupuncture for a minimum cost or for no charge. You can contact an acupuncture college through the British Acupuncture Council and receive treatment from the students under supervision. Otherwise, as with a counsellor, get a good recommendation.

DAY 5

Surrender

Today's task is to surrender to your depression and to write about it. As you surrender, write down what it is you are surrendering. Make a list of three things that you are giving up on in order to surrender to your depression. For example:

- I'm giving up on trying to make myself feel better
- I'm giving up on trying to get him/her to love me
- I'm giving up on trying to change my parents

Once you have identified three things that you are giving up on, write them out on a piece of paper (or use a code) and stick them in front of your nose so that you remember to give them up. Add this entreaty to your day by asking this of your Higher Power:

Grant me the serenity
To accept the things I cannot change,
The courage to change the things I can,
And the wisdom to know the difference.

Recite this as you look at your three things that you are giving up on today.

WRITE A JOURNAL ENTRY

Take 15 minutes to write down your thoughts and feelings. Just let them flow, but head towards the centre of your depression. Write down the deepest pain that you feel today.

WALK OUT TO THE WORLD

Imagine yourself as an island. Imagine everyone else as an island too. We all live together in a large sea. We are separate, but we affect each other. The water between us is affected by what we do and how we react. We need things from other islands in order to survive. But we don't necessarily need it from our closest island – there are many islands we can choose from. We can build bridges to other islands. We don't need to build a bridge to the islands we can see. We can make our bridges stretch out as far as we want to reach an island that has what we need. There are many islands that will delight in our arrival on their beach. We have many choices.

When we are depressed, we often choose to cut ourselves off because we feel ashamed of our depressed feelings. We become isolated, frightened and lonely. When someone passes our island, we smile and wave and pretend we're OK, but under our breath we mutter, 'Bugger off.' And, as soon as they are gone, we stop smiling and hope they don't come back. We have tricked them; they have gone and we have won.

But we haven't won and we feel worse. Our island needs supplies to flourish and ours is looking dry and undernourished. It is dying in the middle but it's only now that it's beginning to show as the leaves start to turn brown and the trees droop with thirst. We need to build a bridge to others for supplies but we're too angry, too sad and too stubborn.

Intimacy is the way that the inner, isolated part of us comes out and feels part of our magnificent world. It is the way that we can feel an integral part of life. It is one way to help us beat depression. Intimacy is the inner part of us connecting with the outer world. When we talk of intimacy, we don't mean a sexual intimacy; we mean intimacy as a way of feeling that we have reached shared ground with another person in a way that is unique to us both. It is the common denominator of two people who have taken a decision to get the conditions right to be honest to the core with each other.

We start building a bridge with a brick. When we are ready, we put down another brick. Start by taking one risk today – just one. Tell someone with whom you want to build a bridge that you feel depressed. Check out your closest friends first. Don't push yourself when it doesn't feel safe, and leave if it feels abusive, but otherwise hang on in there when you just feel like running. It is scary but there is always a back door.

If you have no one to talk to, consider organising a counsellor. See 'Getting Help' in Part 1 for more information on this.

A counsellor is a fast-track route to getting the conditions right for reclaiming our life. Essentially we are paying for someone to:

- listen to us
- acknowledge how we feel
- reflect back how they see it
- help us to work out the solution

For some of us, entering into counselling is akin to paying for the parenting we never received. This is why it is imperative we find someone who won't abuse us further. Again, the previous section under 'Getting Help' will assist us in minimising these risks.

Whether we talk to people we know or seek a professional to help us, we start to establish the first bridge to another island – and this will open doors that we never knew were possible. Things are never as bad as we think they are when we are depressed. This will be confirmed to us when we ask someone else to look at it from his or her perspective.

So, just for today, we find one person to talk to. It can be as simple as responding honestly to someone when they ask, 'How are you?' Instead of saying, 'Fine,' we can say, 'You know, I feel really low today.' We can gauge the response and continue or stop accordingly. We can be prepared to protect ourselves if necessary. Or we can need nothing else but simply to voice to one other person how we are. It may be enough, just for today.

DAY 6
Surrender

If being asked to take a risk is too overwhelming, take a step back and revert to Day 1. Simply surrender to the crushing effect of your depression. This is in respect of yourself. Don't push; you have pushed for too long. Don't demand; you have insisted for too long. Kick back and surrender.

WRITE A JOURNAL ENTRY

Today, write a diary of your food. Simply write down everything you have eaten. Oh, and don't forget all those little bits and pieces you think don't count. At the end of the day, check out your food intake against how you feel. (Remember, this is in addition to your 15-minute daily journal entry.)

DEVELOPING YOUR FAITH

'Faith is the strength by which a shattered world shall emerge into the light' HELEN KELLER

Developing a faith in something will help you get better quicker by developing your trust. No matter how cynical we are, we are all better off with more trust and less control in our lives.

A big part of our depression often stems from our wanting to control other people and outcomes. Until we learn this is not conducive to our wellbeing, we stay stuck. In fact, recovery from depression comes quicker if we learn to control less. However, in order to control less we need to have something else to believe in. What we need to know is that if we let go of control, it will be OK.

What does letting go entail? It means letting go of trying to hold on for dear life to things in spite of knowing that it is killing us!

What do we hold on to? We may try to hold on to another person, unwilling to let them go because we are scared of being alone. We may be trying to hang on to a lifestyle that we can no longer afford or keep up because we are frightened what others might say. We hold on to what is familiar for fear of facing change.

But what is the alternative? For many of us, self-control and control of others has got us nowhere except up a dark alley. Some of us have never lived any other way and have depended on our self-reliance to protect us. We have been taught to be self-sufficient at any cost and to trust that only we can help ourselves.

But the downside is that we feel lonely, resentful and hopeless. We may appear confident but we are aloof or secretive, keeping others away from us because it is too painful to let anyone know how we really feel. We struggle in relationships and need to rely on medicating our feelings to lessen the pain.

It is when our backs are against the wall that we are perhaps at the point where we are most open to change. Putting in place an idea that we can rely on something other than ourselves will help us to free ourselves of the burden of depression. Relying only on ourselves keeps us stuck in the pain of depression, but reaching out in the belief that something other than our self-control can help us will enable us to liberate ourselves.

So, what or who can we turn to?

FAITH IN A GOD

If you have a belief in a God then this should be an easy step for you. Using your confidence, start to turn to God and allow yourself to be guided by Him. Start your day with the following prayer:

I turn my will and my life over to you.
Show what is your wish for me
And how to deliver it in my life, just for today.

With these thoughts uppermost in your mind, you can start to let go a little. Instead of getting frustrated about something you cannot manage, take a deep breath and 'hand it over'. Instead of trying to push the boulder uphill, stand aside and let nature take its course, allowing it to roll down the hill. Allow the love of God to enter you, nourish and heal you.

Letting go of control and letting a God take over doesn't mean we abdicate our responsibilities. It doesn't mean we don't bother to work any more or wait for God to hand us Saturday night's lottery numbers. It means we 'plan but don't project'; we have aims with objectives but we don't force the result; we ask for what we need but we don't demand that someone else does it. We become clear about what we want and then hand it over to our God.

If we allow our faith to develop and grow we will begin to create an inner home to which we will be able to turn when we need warmth and comfort. We will gradually feel the need to control others and outcomes less. We will start to feel more secure in the knowledge that there is a bigger picture than we realise; one over which we have very little influence. We begin to need less control over things, as our faith grows stronger. We become less needy and therefore less frightening to others because we have created a little haven into which we can dive for nourishment. People will come towards us and offer gifts that we may choose or not choose to accept. In time, they will want to know what it is we have and want some for themselves.

No one can violate this sanctuary and our trust will manifest itself as an aid to recovering from depression.

FAITH IN A HIGHER POWER

A Higher Power is any power that is greater than us. There are many perspectives on this idea and here are a few:

- There is the idea of a Universal Law. The Transcendental Meditation movement talks about the power of 'Natural Law'. This is the 'Karmic Law' that maintains that what you give out you will get back. Statements about this power infiltrate our everyday life. We hear statements like 'She's got it coming to her,' or 'What you reap you sow,' or 'I leave it up to fate.' When I look back on my own 'hell on earth' as my husband was going through treatment for cancer, we had two children, no money and no hope. I thought it would never end and I also thought that he would die. Some days I was beside myself with anxiety and grief. I hit a rock bottom and had nowhere else to go but to pray to a Higher Power for help. It didn't seem fair that we should go through this torture. We had harmed no one and couldn't see why this was happening to us. In time my husband recovered and our life returned to a more normal existence. The way I was able to ground myself throughout this time was to write – and hence this book was born. I know that I couldn't have written it without going through what I did: not only for the experiences but also for the escapism it brought me. I can now see it as the Universal Law at work, even though I would have preferred not to go through what I did to produce it.

- There is the power of 'more than one'. Sharing some deep thoughts or feelings with someone we trust can be a powerful experience. When we create an intimate exchange we take a risk and share ourselves with someone and this gives us a feeling of belonging. There is a power that comes with intimacy that can only be generated with two or more people.

It's the power of a group and it's a case of one and one making ten. This creative field is immensely powerful.

- There is faith in fate. This is the idea, 'What will be, will be.' This is a great, pragmatic approach to belief in a Higher Power because we cannot control the future. No matter how skilled we are at making plans they often go awry, much to our frustration. 'Fate' in this sense is a power greater than ourselves and can be relied on as a safety net to help us let go and trust more.

FAITH IN OURSELVES

When we choose to bow out and surrender, the human psyche holds the most powerful means of repairing itself. Like a well-managed ecosystem, we have powers we don't know exist until we put them to the test.

If we allow the natural progression to take place, our spirit will heal itself. If we stop blocking the process of human healing, we will recover from any form of depression we suffer. If we take away the tools that we use to medicate ourselves we allow the natural phenomena of self-recovery to take place. Like the pilot who is in a muddle in his Cessna, if he lets go and trusts, the plane will even out its wings, rudder and nose and fly on an even keel. In other words, we need to get our outer conditions right and let our natural healing take place.

But we have to allow ourselves to review our past – what we have lost and denied we've lost. We have to make sense of our traumas and experience them to shed the blockages they have created. When we experience this two or three times, we will come to realise that we can trust our inner method of restoration because we will feel so much better for unburdening ourselves. We will begin to uncurl, our stomachs will be less tense and we will see sideways, not just ahead.

Another side to having faith in ourselves is to look at our Adult self. We often know what is good for us, what we need, and how to get it. The part of us that knows this is the quiet intellect that resides in the top of us. It is the mental aptitude we have for instinctively knowing the answer. If we learn to sit quietly (explained in Day 13 under Meditation) and ask a question, we can hear the right answer. For some of us it can take some time to refine this technique, but it is available to all of us.

Once we have experienced this depth of knowledge that sits in us, it can feel quite scary to know that we have the answers within ourselves. We can use this part of us for our good, and harness the extraordinary powers we have to help us recover from depression. Faith, whether in God, a Higher Power or our own psyche, does not happen overnight. It is a long journey, but it is the road to freedom. Faith will come as we receive evidence that it works. As we begin to let go of our self-control, things will happen and mini-miracles will arise.

To help us on the journey of recovery, we need to feel that there is something more powerful that can help put us back together. This is why we need faith in something other than ourselves, and yet this can be the hardest part: letting something other than us lend us its help.

MEETING OUR HIGHER POWER

For the sake of simplicity, we shall call whatever we believe in, be it God, our Adult self, the Natural Law, etc., a 'Higher Power'. Below is a visualisation that can help you to meet your Higher Power. This is a very powerful exercise that can be done at any time and as many times as you want. Read this visualisation into a tape, pausing where there are dots and speaking slowly and clearly. Be gentle when you record it and, if you have some favourite music that soothes you, play it in the background as you speak the words. The whole visualisation will take up to twenty minutes.

Start your tape...

This exercise is to help you to meet your Higher Power. Sit or lie down in a comfortable, safe place. Make sure you can lie back and relax. Now simply breathe in and out and let yourself sink into your chair or bed. Thoughts will come into your mind ... do not fret, simply let them float away as quietly as they arrived ... just let them go ... do not hold on to them ... notice your breath coming in and out of your body ... be aware of it travelling through your nose or mouth ... take a deep breath and hold it ... hold it ... hold it more ... keep holding it ... and let it go ... and, as it goes, feel your body completely relax ... notice the worry lines in your forehead relax and soften ... see how your jaw line loosens and your cheek muscles just drop ... feel your throat relax and let the tension out of your chest cavity ... feel the muscles of your stomach drop and relax ... feel the whole weight of your body sink into your chair ... you have no worries or cares right now ... let them drift away with your thoughts ... you are in a lush, green forest ... smell the forest smell and see the damp green blanket sprinkled with sunbeams ... you are on the edge of a river ... this river is beautiful ... it is long and wide and as still as a mirror ... there is a boat by the side of the river ... step into this boat ... it has big, sumptuous pillows for you to sink into ... make yourself comfortable ... you hardly have time to settle and the boat starts to move very gently ... it is gliding along as a gentle swan ... it is being guided and you have nothing to fear ... just sit back and enjoy the beauty of your surroundings ... don't worry if you cannot see them, just get a sense of being there ... all you can hear is the gentleness of trickling water as your boat moves along the flat river ... sit back and relax and feel the moment with no cares and no worries ... in the distance you can see land ... there is a beautiful island ahead of you ... the boat is heading towards the island ... it feels very peaceful and the nearer you get to the island, the more peaceful you feel ... you reach the island and step out of the boat ... there is a mist over the island ... it feels very safe ... it is the most beautiful place you have ever seen ... you are mesmerised by the beauty of the forest, the sound of water, the humming of the trees … you feel safer than you have ever felt before … you breathe in the crisp air and let yourself relax, down … down … down … down into the safety of this island … you see a light in the distance … the light is tiny and just shines through the mist … you can see it moving towards you … as it gets closer, you can feel the energy coming from the light … you can feel a beauty inside you … the light is getting brighter now and the size is much greater … as the light gets closer, it's growing and growing and the energy you can feel from this light is like the love you have always longed for … this feeling is filling you up and the circle of light is now the same size as you … the brightness is beautiful and the beauty is filling every part of your body … the light is right before you … there are messages coming to you from the light … 'You are a beautiful person and I love you more than life itself' … 'I will always love you and protect you' … your Higher Power's love fills you up even more … walk towards the light and step into the light until it surrounds you … let the warmth and love fill you up even more … relax your stomach muscles to allow the love into every part of you … drink the love and let everything else go … nothing else matters right now … fall into the arms of this love and light … speak to your Higher Power and have a conversation with your Higher Power … … … … … [take some time for this] … … … now, step back from the light and let the love stay with you … now your Higher Power has a message for you … hold your hands out and allow your Higher Power to give you a ball of light … take this light into your hands … there is a message on the ball … read it and, when you have finished, gently let the ball go upwards and float away … it is time to leave this island … step into the boat and let it guide you back to the forest … know that you can come back to meet your Higher Power at any time you want … I will count to three and on three you will wake up feeling refreshed, loved and at peace …one, two, three.

Stop your tape

DAY 7
Surrender

This is the seventh day on which we surrender. We will be feeling a new power due to our surrendering. We have gained confidence because we did not fall apart when we surrendered. We have a new strength because we don't need to 'hang on for dear life' as we once thought we did. We have let go and have fallen into the hands of a Higher Power. We have found a freedom that means we don't need to be pretend to ourselves that we are OK when we feel depressed, or treat ourselves with contempt when we feel like a failure because we are depressed.

Just for today, surrender and relish the honesty of your own openness.

WRITE A JOURNAL ENTRY

Write a passage about how it feels to have surrendered for at least seven days in a row. Write about what you are left with. Perhaps it is the nothingness, the utter loneliness or the hopelessness. This is what you have been running from. But it doesn't need to be 'sorted' or 'fixed' or put right just yet. You are facing your fears. There is a way out and that comes in the next seven days. But, for now, simply surrender for this last day and write about it. This will help to settle scores with your self and re-address the balance.

WRITE ABOUT YOUR ANGER

Getting angry is a vital pinnacle in our recovery. There is no doubt that we have swallowed anger and this has made us depressed. Swallowed anger is the main reason for our depression and it's time to address it.

For many of us, if we had expressed our original anger, we would not have become depressed. Many of us struggle to express anger. It is the most common feeling with which we all have difficulty. But there is a straight path through this maze and we can start by writing about who we are angry with.

Take out your journal and write about who you are angry with. If you read this and deny that you're angry with anyone, make no mistake: you are in denial. Depression develops through blocked emotions and anger is the main one. This doesn't mean that another person is responsible for the way you feel. It means that you have swallowed some anger about something or someone and you have not allowed yourself to express it. You can begin the process of finding out what you have suppressed by writing about it.

The great thing about our journal is that we can start off by blaming the world and no one will need to see it. At a later date we can unravel the blame and take responsibility for what we haven't put in place to protect ourselves. But, for now, we will simply write about our anger as a child would – full of blame and self-pity because, if we are depressed, it is in there somewhere, and there is no better place to get it out than into our private journal.

We have come to the end of our first Seven Days

The first seven days of surrender is to help us come into ourselves and give up on trying to control the uncontrollable outside world. It is about grounding us and closing the focus in on ourselves. This will help us to redirect our energy into healing ourselves.

It is important not to go past Day 7 until you feel that you have reclaimed your concentration and used it to create a personal hub. You will be sure that you have been saturated by this stage because you will become frustrated and bored. This makes it easier for us to stop running away from our fears and harnesses our power to help us overcome them. It's akin to stepping off a roller coaster that has depleted us of all our energy, because we have been trying to hang on for our life. By stepping off the ride, we can rest up and build strength to have a look at where we have come from.

The next part of this 14-day plan is to help us focus on where we are headed to now, and how we are going to work ourselves towards reclaiming our life.

DAY 8

Surrender No More

'Are you in earnest? Seize this very minute!
Boldness has genius, power, and magic in it.
Only engage, and then the mind grows heated.
Begin, and then the work will be completed.'

JOHN ANSTER

When we have held ourselves back, after a given amount of
time we naturally start to feel frustrated. This frustration is the
catalyst to our next move. We surrender no more, but begin to
experience the power that comes when we have shed enough
pain and freed ourselves up to take better care of ourselves.

WRITE IT OUT

The next task goes one step further in reclaiming your life.
It is primarily for those of us who don't understand why we
are depressed, or else we know why we are depressed but
don't understand why it affects us so badly.

Within every exchange that we have, we play a part – and we
have a responsibility for the part we play. If we are depressed,
the part we play can seem far removed from the reality, and we
feel controlled or manipulated by others and other situations.
In reclaiming our life, we have to ascertain our part, identify
our responsibility, and become accountable. This next section
aims to address this.

When we are depressed we may interact with others in a
'neurotic' way. In many cases we will choose to play the Victim,

Perpetrator or Martyr/Rescuer. These roles are tied up together so that we find we switch from one to another at a moment's notice. Sometimes we feel we have no power over this – it just happens and we can't understand why. These roles are explained as follows:

- As victims we feel as though we have no power and no choices. We are at the mercy of others and we cannot take our own decisions. We discount ourselves and prefer others to see us as having no influence. We feel ignored, we feel hopeless and we feel helpless. We also feel tremendous shame for having these feelings.

- As perpetrators we feel angry about being the victim and we believe that others have made us like this, so we turn on them. We are enraged at the way others treat us and, consequently, we don't want anyone near us. We make sure that no one gets in our way. We behave abusively by turning our self-abuse onto others. We can see that we frighten others and, even though we are remorseful, it doesn't stop us.

- As martyrs/rescuers we look at the 'victim' and feel it is our duty to rescue them, whether they want it or not! We do things for others or rescue them because we want something back – but we don't tell them what it is. Underneath our 'good deeds' we are waiting to get noticed and get our rewards. Let's face it, what would they do without us? It is our job to keep others together. If it wasn't for us they wouldn't survive. When we don't receive our reward we then turn back into the victim and feel helpless, hopeless and futile once more.

With depression, we lose the ability to be objective. We tend to gravitate to one or more of these roles. I have acted out all three in one day – many times! The cycle of depression keeps us stuck in these roles and we find it near impossible to step away from them. The more difficult we find it, the more likely it is that we were taught these roles as children. But even though these roles are comfortable and familiar, they hold us back from recovering from depression. We need to take a look at them.

These questions address these issues. You may not be able to answer them promptly. Don't concern yourself with a timescale but respond to them when you know the answers.

The path out of these neurotic ways of thinking is telling the truth. We have to begin by delving deep and asking ourselves what is our true motivation behind our behaviour? What is it we want when we take on the mantle of the victim, persecutor or martyr? We don't really want to feel helpless and hopeless and to be seen like this. Given the choice, we would prefer to feel liberated, blissful and excited about being alive.

This next exercise can help you to grab the essence of the behaviour that drives you round in circles and give you some answers for how to change. The more honest you can be, the more informative the results will be.

These are the questions you must ask yourself:

1 When have I had these feelings before?

Depression is caused by 'de-pressed' feelings; feelings which have been pressed down. When this happens, the depression races in and fills the space left by the pressed-down feelings. But these feelings are not so far away. This question relates to the pressed-down feelings. Grab them and draw them out. When have I experienced them before?

When did they start? Put three memories to the experiences. Find a photo that symbolises the timing of the feelings or visualise yourself at the time that you were previously depressed. How often do I experience them?

Do I experience them in the company of someone I hardly know? Or is it only with certain members of my family or friends?

2 What triggers their reoccurrence?

Who or what triggers these feelings?

What situation do I get myself into that triggers these feelings?

Why does it always happen when I go to work/ visit my brother/ argue with my wife? (Find your own situation.)

3 Which role do I play in this situation i.e. victim, martyr or perpetrator?

Which role do I play in this situation?

Why do I take up this role?

How long have I been playing this part?

If I become the victim, then who is the perpetrator?

Who taught me this role? Or from whom did I learn it?

4 What benefits do I gain from being here?

Why do I play this part?

What is my payoff?

Who am I trying to please? And why?

5 By playing this part, what am I trying to avoid?

What situation am I trying to avoid by playing this part?

What feelings do I avoid when I play this part?

What is it in myself that I am circumnavigating when I am in this role?

6 What are the roles that others are playing?

Who do I see as the perpetrator?

If I am the perpetrator, who is my victim?

If I am the martyr, who am I rescuing?

7 What do I need to do to change this?

If I had no fear of anyone doing anything threatening to me, and no negative outcome was possible, what would be an ideal scenario for me to make changes that benefit me? This is an opportunity to map out your best-case scenario to help you recover from depression. For example, when I was depressed I wanted someone to come along and just take care of me and all my problems. I wanted someone to deal with my perceived enemies, take care of my son, give me enough money to live on, offer me a brilliant job and tell me I was OK. Just write your own perfect setting with lots and lots of details. Embellish it until it becomes a perfect picture for you. Take your time – hours, days, weeks. Don't rush this important bit. Get all the detail down and see it in your mind's eye.

Once you have outlined your best-case scenario, imagine yourself to be in front of a panel of the top five people that you most admire. These can be people that you personally know or people you have never met but for whom you have great respect. Ask each of them this question: 'What do I have to do to get my best case scenario to come true?'

Write down each answer as it comes to you. When they have answered, savour the results, because within this exercise we can be sure we are accessing the best of ourselves. The answers are now in our hands and we know what we need to do next.

DAY 9

Surrender No More

It's now time to purge yourself of your 'victim' status.

When we are depressed, we feel that we are victims of many things: society, another's control, authority, our parents' behaviour, personal finances, our workplace, etc. This is because we have felt powerless – a debilitating state of mind that can paralyse us, and from which we feel we have no refuge. We can't even see why this is happening to us and we beg for help, we pray for mercy, or we look to others to help us get out of the mire. When we feel we have no choices, it can feel as though we are sinking into a bog from which we can't escape.

We have to acknowledge that we were once victims but, as we gain strength and self-responsibility, we are victims no more. If we suffer from feeling like a victim, this was probably due to a legacy from our childhood. Those of us who were raised without feeling a sense of autonomy will often carry this feeling into adulthood, and it will seep into our everyday life.

It will manifest itself as a feeling of dependence on others to survive. Becoming aware of our 'victim' status is the first step towards changing it.

We are not alone in this thinking. Our society is entrenched in the 'victim' culture. We are steeped in the idea that other people have a much bigger influence over us than is actually correct. We hear it in conversations, songs, fiction, the media, etc. We hear people constantly living out the victim culture: 'I can't live without you', 'She made me do it', 'You're holding me back', 'My life is incomplete without you', 'He makes me feel terrible about myself', etc.

As a nation, we live in a huge fantasy that constantly plays itself out, and we have been suckered into it. There comes a time when we have to purge ourselves of this propaganda to help us beat depression.

Some myths to be demolished:

- Someone else is responsible for the way we feel.

  It is not possible for another person to get inside us and change the way we feel. We put ourselves in situations that have an effect on us. It is our responsibility. Someone will say something to three people and the effect that it has on those three people will differ. What effect another person's words has on us is down to our own thinking, beliefs etc. No one can put you down without your permission.

- We can expect 'unconditional love' from another adult.

  Actually, we can't. Unconditional love from one adult to another is unrealistic. Many relationships with others are based on one party demanding this from another. This may easily lead to us feeling very depressed because we can end up feeling unworthy if we have based our ideals on someone else loving us 'no matter what'. Every adult relationship has a contract, whether written or unwritten. For instance, many couples would not tolerate one partner having an affair. Whether this is written down or not, it is understood.

If we enter into a relationship expecting 'unconditional love', we are entering into it with a child's outlook. We cannot contemplate a fulfilling adult relationship until we have finished our childhood. If we try to build a relationship before we have finished our childhood, we are setting ourselves up to take up the victim status.

- She/he made me do it.

Our victim culture pushes us to believe that others have power over us and can make us do things we don't want to, stay in relationships we don't want to be in, and so on. Of course, this is totally false. No one can make us do something we don't wish to do. The exception is when the other person is breaking the law by blackmailing us or holding a gun to our head – an extremely unlikely scenario. But when we hear ourselves saying, 'They made me do it,' we have to ask ourselves: was there a gun at my head at the time? In fact, no one has that much power over us unless we simply give it away.

- Others have control over us.

Other people have control over us only when we let them. This is usually because we want something back from them. Again, the only exception to this is if someone is breaking the law by using violence or holding us against our will.

- We have control over others.

It is arrogant of us to believe we have so much power that we can control others. Indeed, if someone is allowing us to control them, it's time to look at why they would do that. What are they receiving in return, and do we want a relationship that includes us being in control of another?

- I can't live without him/her.

Yes you can. If this is your thinking, it is time to see what is so frightening about being independent and why you are hiding behind someone else for comfort.

The following exercises will start to help you unravel some of the mysteries that come with living in the Victim Culture.

TAKING ON RESPONSIBILITY

'Our discontent begins by finding false villains whom we can accuse of deceiving us. Next we find false heroes who we expect to liberate us. The hardest, most discomfiting discovery is that each of us must emancipate himself.'

DANIEL J. BOORSTIN

WHO DO WE GIVE OUR POWER TO?

If we think someone has power over us, we are misguided. If someone has power over us it is because we allow it. If we are afraid of someone, it is because we have given up our power. If they 'rule us' it is because we let them. If we obey them then it is because we get a payoff.

If we stay in a difficult relationship, the payoff may be that we rely on our partner for financial or practical support, or we can't face being on our own. We may not confront the difficulties because we don't want to rock the boat and face the possible consequences of the boat rocking. If we rely on our partner to support us, then we're scared of going out into the world to find ways of supporting ourselves. If we rely on our partner to be our 'other half', it's because we are scared of being alone.

These scenarios, and many more, are about our inability or refusal to grow up, take responsibility for ourselves and take care of ourselves as adults. We are acting as children who need A.N. Other to be our parent. We are relying on another adult to care for us and protect us because we actually think we can't do it for ourselves. We weave ourselves into the guise of a 'good' relationship with our protector, to whom we have given up our power in order that we may be taken care of.

We have mapped out an unspoken contract that works well in terms of who does what and what the whole team achieves. We have probably done this without any considered plan – it just happened.

What are the consequences?

We have to give up a lot in order to maintain the stability of the power contest. We may allow ourselves to be bullied, neglected, shamed, and physically or sexually abused. We may stop ourselves from reaching our own potential in terms of a career or creative pursuit. We might sabotage our friendships to please our partner.

We become blinkered to other opportunities. This is driven by fear – fear of others and fear of the unknown. Many of us who have suffered from depression have given our power away – often in ignorance – and this has led us down a long and painful path. This is the time to readjust the power balance.

How do we readjust the power balance?

This exercise will help you identify how and why we hand power over and how you can start to reclaim it.

1   In your journal, write down the main person you have in your mind while reading this section.
2   Write down 3 examples of what you do when you are with them that you would rather you didn't do.
3   Write down why you act like this.
4   How does it affect you when you compromise yourself?
5   What is the feeling of loss? What feelings or issues are you sidestepping?
6   What do your feelings remind you of?
7   If you turned away from that person with these feelings intact, what would you do to resolve your dilemma?
8   And what practical action could you take?

A very common reason why someone is depressed is that they hold on to a relationship that is not right for them because they are very frightened of being single. We can feel so 'close' to another that the thought of being without them can send us into a panic. The ongoing compromising we do to maintain a relationship can be at a great cost to ourselves. Indeed, the greater our fear of being alone, the greater our need to compromise ourselves, and the more power we give to another.

If we give our power away to another person in a close relationship, the chances are we also still hold our parents in an authoritative place. If we view our parents as adults and as equals, we are less likely to 'cling' to another to avoid being on our own. For this reason, it may be wise to address our relationship with our parents before we move out of our partner's pad and fall apart without him/her.

The fastest way of addressing our issues with other people is to identify what it is we are frightened of confronting, e.g. getting a job, being on our own, meeting new people, and look at how we are using another person to shield us from our fears.

WE NEED TO ASK OURSELVES THESE QUESTIONS:

- **What is it about this person that I imagine they are 'doing something' to me?**
- **What do I do to compromise myself in their company?**
- **What is it I am so afraid of that I am willing to compromise what I really want to do/think/see/feel by hiding behind them?**

If we can ask ourselves these questions and start writing a piece in our journal every day, we will find the end of the ball of wool and begin to unravel a mystery that can lead to new insights – and these insights will help us to reclaim our life. This exercise will act like a hot knife through butter. The more we work on it, the more we will balance our relationships, because we will naturally compromise ourselves less.

Remember, this is learned behaviour. No one is born with a goal to feel like a victim or suffer depression. This route to identifying what keeps us feeling 'stuck' in a relationship is a good starting point.

In your journal, write down a list of people to whom you give your power. Work out how you will readjust the power balance. You can be assured that there is no quick fix and that this is a lifelong exercise. But the awareness you gather from undertaking these first steps is a lifelong tool and will help you with every area of your life. You will be on your way to beating your depression.

❊ ❊ ❊

DAY 10
Surrender no more

While staying with the momentum of recovery from depression, it is a good time for us to identify what triggers our depressed feelings. As we start to move away from feeling chronically depressed, we can become aware of what situations hook us back into that sinking, hopeless feeling that we are so used to. Our recovery is fragile to start with, but we build strength day by day.

If we take our journal and write out what scenarios push us backward, we can then be aware of them, and either avoid those situations or arm ourselves so we are prepared. Simply knowing what our triggers are will help us halfway towards conquering difficult circumstances.

- **Returning to the parental home**
- **Work appraisals**
- **Eating junk food**
- **Christmas**
- **Receiving an 'overdue for payment' letter**
- **Being rejected when asking someone on a date**
- **Husband/wife refusing sex**
- **Bingeing on drink and/or drugs**
- **A 'look' from an authority**
- **Self-recrimination**
- **Lack of exercise**

When we are aware of our triggers we have choices. Choices offer us a new power and a new road to reclaiming our life.

DIVIDE INTO THREE

'At the innermost core of all loneliness is a deep and powerful yearning for union with one's lost self.' **BRENDAN FRANCIS**

We are made up of a variety of components. The components encompass emotions, morals, voices spinning around our head, values, principles, ethics, a 'right and wrong' agenda, suppressed feelings, out of control feelings, opinions, beliefs, hidden agendas, plans, schedules, motivations, competitions to win, struggles to maintain, lies to cover up and judgements to be made. And, when we are depressed, we can feel as though we are losing the 'plot', especially when others tell us to sort ourselves out! Where do we start to help ourselves?

If there is one method that is accessible to everyone, it is the 'Divide Into Three' approach that I spoke about in the section 'Five Things To Do When Your Head Is Above Water' (Suggestion 9). In our psyche, there lives our Child self, our Parent self and our Adult self. The Child holds our emotions. The Parent holds the parenting rules we have learned from our own parents. The Adult is the link to our God, our Higher Power.

THE CHILD

For some of us, the mere mention of the 'child' in us can make us cringe and run for cover. We are frightened by the thought of uncovering this part of us. We are ashamed of this part of us because it is where we store our secrets, the things we would never tell anyone else, the habits we carry out which, if anyone else were to see, we would die of embarrassment. But the Child in us also carries our pain, stores our anger and obeys the rules which say they are too shameful or too painful to be let out.

Children are naturally joyful. If we look around at children at play, they are laughing, shouting, exploring and screaming with delight. For those of us who are depressed, joy can mean an absence of depression, an absence of pain or no feelings at all. But true joy is what children express when they're happy. Their behaviour is a good indicator of where we want to be.

The Child in us holds our emotions. The Child obeys the rules, and if the rules are 'don't talk, don't trust, don't feel', then the Child will do what the rules say and stay blocked and depressed. However, we have the potential to feel as joyful as those children we see playing with their friends.

THE ADULT

The Adult is our wisdom. Knowledge can be taught but wisdom cannot. We are born with this wisdom. This wisdom has no grievance, nor ignorance. Our wisdom knows the proper limits for ourselves. Our wisdom can distinguish between good and evil. It can weigh up all significant factors, get a sense of proportion, and attach importance to a problem. Our wisdom has no fear, grief, malice or arrogance. Our wisdom is our clean self. Our wisdom is the part of us that knows the truth even if we don't want to hear it.

The Adult is the part of us that is linked to our Higher Power. This part of us can access our true path and holds the information we need to be loyal to ourselves. We can start to listen to this part of us and trust what we hear. We can call on our Adult at any time for the right answer.

It may take some time to get the hang of this technique but it will come. It took me several years to hear my Adult voice, and that was because I constantly dismissed it as nonsense. I didn't trust myself enough, but meditation helped me – as well as doing the exercise to meet my Higher Power (see Day 6 – 'Developing Your Faith'). I now find the answers come quickly.

THE PARENT

The Parent is the part of ourselves that governs us. It has absorbed rules and regulations and has passed these on to the Child. The messages we hear from the Parent can be loving, gentle and affirming or harsh, critical and judgemental. Our Parental messages will have been put in place by how we were parented as children. It's not often we get a chance to challenge these rules but this is a good time to begin.

If we are depressed, it will have a lot to do with feeling under pressure to live by someone else's values. If we had challenged the authority of others, we might not be depressed now. We would also have a Parent who is present to take care of the Child in a way that engendered self-responsibility, joy, fun and satisfaction. But we don't, so this is the time to have a look at how the Parent treats us and make changes that will help us beat depression and reclaim our life.

The Negative Parent

To start to hear the Parent in us, we can make this statement: 'I want to put everything down and go out to play.' Listen hard to the voice that follows the statement. For those of us who are depressed, the voice will usually sound critical and put up a barrier. For example, 'There is too much to do,' 'This is no time to play,' or 'You've no right to start demanding pleasure at a time like this.' We might find that the voice sounds exactly like that used by our parents when we were children. The more we delve into the parental voices, the clearer it becomes. In time we find that we can spot this voice in an instant. It doesn't take long to develop this skill. Within three days of consistently listening to the internal criticism, we will have good clues to which voice is negatively parenting us.

The Loving Parent

There is a loving Parent inside us as well as a negative Parent. We want to mobilise the loving Parent for our good. We can identify this loving Parent when we hear the soothing voice or the 'pat on the back' voice. It may seem hard to grasp this to begin with and if we struggle with this part of ourselves, we can actually 'borrow' someone else's loving Parent for a moment.

To do this, we do something for someone else and wait for their response. If we help a short person by reaching for an item off the top shelf, let a harassed parent go first in the queue, or help an older person along the road, we will get a positive response. Then we can feel what it's like to experience a warm glow in our stomach – the Child part of us.

With persistence we can start to separate the loving Parent away from the negative Parent and use the loving influence to put pressure on the nagging, critical voice that can dominate us.

For example, what we want to hear in response to, 'I want to put everything down and go out to play' is something like, 'We have work to do for the next two hours but after that we shall go out for a walk; we can fit it in before we have to make dinner.' The Child in us wants fairness and support. We have to acknowledge that we need to have some nurturing time in order to feel whole and loved.

If you've been depressed for a long time, you may have lost the gist of what you need to feel un-depressed. Write out a list of five things you would like to do when time is free. Remember – the Child in us doesn't need money to have a good time. Like a child, we want and crave love and attention; that's what will get us feeling good – not the money substitute. And now we can give ourselves love and attention because we have the tools and the know-how.

The loving Parent will also manage the Child by setting limits, being fair and firm, listening and explaining, talking the Child through fear, and making decisions for the best. For those of us who find these parameters difficult to grasp, we can get help in order that we learn how to do this. We can watch people speaking to their children and learn from this. We can enrol on parenting courses. We can seek counselling.

Most profound, however, is to ask our own seat of wisdom – our Adult self. This is how the three parts of us work together. The depressed Child turns to the Parent for reassurance, guidance and love, and the Parent turns to the Adult for the correct information to assist the Child to grow up.

The problem is that one doesn't trust the other. The Child doesn't trust the Parent to take care of him, and often with good reason. The Parent doesn't trust the Child not to behave in an appropriate manner. If we believed we were truly adult, we wouldn't feel depressed because the Adult's intellect, reason and logic would take care of our lives and teach us how to parent ourselves in order that the Child part of us can trust the Adult. Our Child needs a stable and reasoned Parent to trust.

This is a central hub of reclaiming our life. So, we need to identify each part of us and help ourselves to function to our potential. How do we do this?

There are many ways we can approach this question and this is covered under 'Divide into Three' in the first section of the book. However, one concise method of separating the child from the parent is to look at how we talk negatively to ourselves.

To begin with, we identify how we negatively parent ourselves in a way that renders us crumpled and depressed. This would include things we say to ourselves:

- You're hopeless
- You can do nothing right
- Why don't you get off your backside and do something
- I hate you when you slump like this
- You should have got over this by now
- Why bother, nobody cares anyway
- You never get it right

Sometimes these phrases are so ingrained in us that we can't even hear them. Remember that nothing keeps us 'pressed down' and blocked like verbal abuse.

'A Native American elder once described his own inner struggles in this manner: "Inside of me there are two dogs. One of the dogs is mean and evil. The other dog is good. The mean dog fights the good dog all the time." When asked which dog wins, he reflected for a moment and replied, "The one I feed the most."'

GEORGE BERNARD SHAW, BRITISH DRAMATIST

LEARN TO TALK TO YOURSELF

This task is about re-parenting ourselves. Re-parenting is simply about finding a new way to talk to ourselves which is supportive, constructive, gentle and firm. This technique is covered in the first part and below is an exercise which will further this development – integration.

Integration

Integration is the bringing together of all parts of us so that we may feel 'whole' or 'complete'. Integration is about tempering the negative Parent, feeding the hungry Child and sourcing the wisdom on how to do this from our Adult.

EXERCISE 1:

Write down all the messages you give out to yourself. The more you listen to yourself, the more you will hear. Just jot them down in your journal and become more aware of them.

EXERCISE 2:

What are you demanding from yourself that the Child part of you is not fulfilling? For example, when I started to listen I discovered that every message I gave myself was critical. I was looking for complete perfection in myself. Decide what is behind your self-criticism and write it in your journal.

EXERCISE 3: AMEND YOUR EXPECTATIONS OF YOURSELF.

In my case, I realised it is not human to demand flawlessness. I am a human being and humans are flawed. Though it has taken me many years to appreciate this in a very profound way, I started the whole journey by amending what I expected of myself and I lowered my demands. This didn't come easy! I had to ask others what they expected of themselves. I had to ask others what they thought of my self-imposed goals. I attended a 12-Step group and listened to other people and their method of 'kicking back' and easing up on themselves. After some months I cautiously began to administer some of this antidote to myself. This helped me because I was allowing myself to be more 'normal' and not the superhuman being that I was scared to let go of. I know now that appearing superhuman was my way of covering up my depression and frailty. It is also a way of keeping others away from me.

By amending our expectations of ourselves, we may begin to raise the anger that has been dormant. This is part of the natural grief process, with the grief being for what we have lost through our self-criticism.

EXERCISE 4:

Taking the negative messages from the first exercise, write next to them a phrase that is nurturing and comforting. Make up Post-it notes, or use codes, and put five of these new messages up around your house or somewhere where you will walk past them and notice them continuously.

For example, the critical messages below now have a new and supportive note next to them:

You're hopeless	You are not hopeless, you are feeling down at the moment but it will pass and you will have more energy to 'do stuff'
You can do nothing right	You do many things right
Why don't you get off your backside and DO something	You are recovering from depression, which is debilitating; easy does it
I hate you when you slump like this	I can sense that you need some time out and I will sort it for you
You should have got over this by now	Depression can take a long time to recover from
Why bother, nobody cares anyway	I care
You never get it right	You get many things right. These include: XYZ

As you see these new messages simply read them to yourself as you walk by. Feel your anger rise as you feel cheated of being yourself. Tell the Parent in you to get stuffed when you hear the continual condemnation. Tell your Parent to go to hell and leave you alone.

At the same time, find your nurturing Adult come out to soothe you. We all want comforting words and touch. We need to treat ourselves with gentleness and love. The Adult is the place to go for new information. If it is reluctant to come to you, ask your Adult for help. Make up your own prayer and say it over and over. Persist with this exercise, because it will eventually come to you.

Some new rules

There are some rules that we can undertake which will help us learn to re-parent ourselves. Some of these rules may replace our old rules. They are as follows:

1 It's OK to make mistakes; this is a normal part of life and making mistakes helps us to learn.
2 Stop lying. Lying causes unnecessary stress in our life because we need to be so vigilant in keeping up the circle of lies. This is a waste of energy.
3 It is OK to feel whatever you feel. Feelings are normal, whatever they are; they are a natural response to life.
4 It is OK and even essential to have fun, go out to play and laugh.
5 It is OK to set boundaries by saying 'NO'. This will help us feel more safe and liberated.
6 It's OK to be different from others.
7 We don't have to compete with others to be good enough.
8 It's imperative that we take responsibility for ourselves and our actions.
9 It is OK to need other people in our life.
10 We no longer have to control others to feel safe. Safety now grows inside us as we take care of ourselves.

As we weed out the critical direction that we give ourselves, we will leave a space for these and other new rules to settle into their place.

We may think that it is someone else who is 'making' us depressed by continually criticising us; there is a well-known assumption that we actually project our own blockages on to the people we are drawn to. This is because when we are stuck, as we are when we are depressed, we are attracted to people who will parallel our inner voice and treat us the way we treat ourselves. This brings the steadfast problem to the fore and causes us to face up to the blockage.

We have to stop blaming other people for our dilemma and take responsibility for our own quandary if we want to beat depression. This can seem so hard when all we can see is another person bullying or victimising us. If we can identify our internal criticism – and our Child's reaction – and find the strength to change it, we can begin to notice the power we have to change our own feelings. Try the exercises in 'Talk To Yourself' and 'One Amazing Thing' in Part 1 of this book. Just try them once to become fully aware of the difference one half-hour can make to the way you feel about yourself.

DAY 11
Surrender No More

It is easy to lose sight of why we have begun this journey.
It is the long road home and it can be painful and frightening,
but illuminating and liberating. We have begun this journey
because we have felt backed up against a wall or we have sunk
into what we thought was a bottomless pit from which there
was no return. Now we are taking ourselves through this
excursion of self-exposure and helping ourselves to emerge
from the darkness and see light again.

Along the way there are many obstacles. The 14-day plan's
tasks are tools to help us clear those obstacles and allow the
natural healing process do its work. We are contaminated with
'toxic waste' that we need to sweep away and the daily tasks
will help us to achieve this. The journey is akin to a canal. The
natural flow of the canal easily becomes blocked with debris
and waste dropped by ourselves and others. These tasks help
us to unlock the canal gates and let the waste flow away.

We surrender no more to the build-up of debris. We use
our new energy to clear the waste. This will give us the tools
we need to climb out of our pit and feel the sun on our spirit.
A vital tool for helping us to do this is to address our anger.

ADDRESS YOUR ANGER

'Anger is a great force. If you control it, it can
be transmuted into a power which can move
the whole world.'

SRI SWAMI SIVANANDA, INDIAN PHYSICIAN, SAGE

Now that we have begun to purge ourselves of our victim mentality and to talk to ourselves with more compassion, we will start to feel safer to allow 'de-pressed' feelings to surface. The most common buried feeling that we have if we are depressed is anger. We started to address our anger by writing about it in our journal on Day 7. It is time to push forward again and confront it more fully.

Anger can be frightening to many of us. The consequence of being around other people's anger may have required us to submerge our own. This is often done to try to appease someone and protect ourselves from something we could not face. This is common in children, where an angry parent is frightening to a child, so we learn to pacify the adult to save ourselves from harm.

However, our own anger is often even more frightening to us. If it wasn't, we wouldn't submerge it and we wouldn't be depressed. I have never met a depressed person who has not buried anger. This is the most common reason for depression.

But anger encompasses many factors. It doesn't just mean seeing ourselves as a raging, screaming banshee! We can feel irritated, frustrated, infuriated, annoyed or snappy. A good indicator of anger is when we don't want much to do with someone we care about. We want to turn away and we don't really know why. For those of us who have been depressed for a long time, we may feel numb when we talk about hidden anger. We can't feel anger because it is just not safe. If you are unsure about whether or not you carry buried anger, there is a 'Checklist For Hidden Anger' in Part 1 (Suggestion 4, 'Get Angry/Cry'). Read through this list to see if you recognise any of the scenarios.

Some of us can be so frightened of expressing anger that it may come out in tears. If we tell ourselves that it is wrong to feel anger, it may be that we feel so guilty, we end up trying to act as though we are sad or hurt. This is manipulative behaviour that we must look at because it compromises us.

However, we have learned to do this to protect ourselves and as we talk to ourselves more, comfort ourselves more and take care of ourselves better, we will feel less guilty for feeling angry and more certain that we have a right to feel angry.

And we do have a right to feel angry. Anger is simply another feeling that is in the same grief cycle as joy, sadness, depression and denial. It's no better or worse. It's just a feeling. The scary part of anger is when it's not expressed, because a build-up of unexpressed anger leads to rage – and we are all capable of madness under the influence of rage. It is time to open the dam that has held back our anger and, little by little, we can let it out until we have a manageable flow.

HISTORIC ANGER

Historic anger is anger that we have not expressed at the time we felt it. This feeling does not simply vanish into thin air when we can't feel it anymore. It has buried itself inside us. It has been said that if we have a consistent feeling for more than 15 minutes, it is historic. If we are depressed, then the chances are pretty good that we hold historic anger.

We witness historic anger being acted out all the time. Road rage is a great example. We know that one person nipping in front of another in their car cannot warrant screaming abuse, assault or murder. Yet it does. The reason for the road rage is that the person who is enraged has a stockpile of historic anger just waiting to explode and, if we are unlucky, we could do something that triggers it.

For some of us the dam described above symbolises the holding back of a huge reservoir of historic anger that surges up behind the wall, trying to get through and making the dam walls strain to the limit. Our psyche has not been prepared to address this anger and has pushed it down, rendering us depressed. We will start to address this anger by the following exercise that will serve to open up a tap on the edge of the dam, allowing a small but measured movement of water to begin.

First, look back over the last year and write down the answers to these questions:

1 What do you feel angry about?
2 With whom do you feel angry?
3 Why do you feel angry?

Answer these three questions as thoroughly as you can in your journal. The answers always appear surprisingly short and succinct. There is usually a very good reason why we are angry and we usually know what that is. We can begin to address this anger now by finding the part of us that is frightened or unsure about addressing the anger. This is the Child part of us. We need to finish off the past and we can do this by undertaking the following exercise.

VISUALISATION EXERCISE

Close your eyes. Visualise yourself in a childlike state and in the company of the person that you are angry with. In this visualisation, see yourself as an adult and take the hand of the child. Stand firm and tall to the person with whom you are angry. As the adult, tell the other person what you both (you and your child) are angry about. You can shout, scream, hurl insults or just talk calmly. Make sure you get the point across until you feel that everything has been said. Ask your child if he would like to say anything. Explain to the other adult that you will not be tolerating their unacceptable behaviour any more. Walk away from that person, holding your child's hand firmly and, when you get to a safe place, bend down to your child and ask if that was OK, and if there was anything more you could have done. Take the child in your arms and tell them you will never, ever let them be steam-rollered by that person again.

When you open your eyes, take in the experience. Whatever you feel, you will know that you can go back to that person and deal with their mistreatment until you feel saturated. The more we undertake this exercise, the more we build up a strong inner core that we will never have experienced before. It is one we can return to.

Write to the person with whom you are angry. Allow your Child to speak this time. Write with your non-usual hand and allow the wretchedness to come out onto paper. Do not send the letter to the person at whom it is directed but, as an exercise for your Child self, address it to a false address (make sure it is a false address), stamp it and post it. Just try this once and feel the satisfaction of it.

This exercise may bring up feelings of anger at all the other people who we have allowed to mistreat us. It may bring up sadness at the way we've allowed ourselves to be abused. Whatever the outcome, this simple exercise will start the whole process of diminishing the powerful and depressive effect that buried anger possesses and is a lifelong tool for dealing with many issues from our past. As we work on our buried anger, the space that comes from releasing old feelings will be filled with a new power. This will help us to fulfil our ability to deal with present anger. The stronger we become, the quicker and gentler we will be in confronting difficult problems in our day-to-day life. This exercise will fast-track our recovery from depression.

PRESENT ANGER

As we lessen the burden of historic anger, we will find it easier to express our anger at something that happens today. Some of us take a long time to get to the point where we can deal with something we don't like as it happens. One of the reasons for this is that we are frightened that we may go out of control. But big anger starts with an irritation and works its way into a large ball. Once we have a handle on the historic anger, expressing present anger will become second nature.

The first thing we must do if we are frightened of expressing ourselves is to take time out when we feel angry. This will give us an opportunity to get a perspective on how angry it is appropriate to feel. We can ask another person to listen to us and help us divide up what is historic anger and what is present anger.

It is best to express our anger as close to the moment as is possible. The sooner we let it out, the easier it is to discharge and the better we feel for it. Anger can mean slight irritation; it doesn't have to mean 'all out war'. However we feel, we are entitled to our feelings. No matter how unreasonable it may sound, if that's how we feel then that's how we feel.

HERE ARE SOME HINTS TO APPROACH EXPRESSING PRESENT ANGER:

- Use plenty of words to express anger that will seem gentler than the word 'angry'. For example: irritated, frustrated, bothered, perturbed, etc.
- Start by expressing anger over trivial things. For example, 'I am frustrated when you don't call when you say you will.'
- Be open to others' responses as they explain their position. For example, they might say, 'I didn't realise that my phone call meant so much to you.' This offers a chance of building a bridge.
- Try to explain what is beneath your anger. For example, 'I am frustrated when you don't call when you say you will because I worry about your wellbeing.'
- Don't express your anger when you are in a state of rage; no one wins at this point.
- As long as you are not in a state of rage, express your anger as soon as you can after the feelings arise.

Practise the words you need to express how you feel when you are alone, or with someone who is neutral and supportive, before you take it to the person for whom the anger is intended.

In terms of expressing anger, practice really does make perfect. At the beginning we find ourselves shaking like a leaf, screaming our heads off or bursting into tears. When we effectively practise expressing our anger, we will feel magnificent because we have found a way to assert ourselves that we can apply to any situation and get good results. We therefore feel that less and less can intimidate us and we feel free to live life with a permanent feeling of lightness.

Sometimes, however, we feel unclear and muddled about a situation and we need to take stock before we respond. A tip for delaying our response is to have to hand a couple of routine phrases that will help us get through those tricky moments when we are flummoxed for what to say. My favourite ones are:

- Thank you for that information, I'll take that away and think about it
- Oh, that's interesting, I didn't know that you saw it that way

This will give us time to evaluate what the other person is saying and to calm ourselves down if we are presented with a situation that renders us incapable of a clear reply. We can then come back to the person and continue where we left off with clarity and good judgement.

The more we practise releasing present anger, the more liberated we feel. As we become more used to expressing anger on the spur of the moment, the less it will burden us and the safer we will feel because we know that we no longer need to run from a situation where we think we can't cope. We can cope, we can say what we need to say, and we can face whatever used to terrify us.

This will play a very big part in beating depression and reclaiming our life.

DAY 12
Surrender No More

'The minute you settle for less than you deserve, you get even less than you settled for.'

MAUREEN DOWD, AMERICAN NEWSPAPER COLUMNIST

Now we are becoming more confident in our ability to release our anger, we can comfortably use it to empower ourselves. This is because we are less afraid of our own anger and have learned to trust ourselves fully when we feel angry. We can use this new-found confidence to restore faith in ourselves that we are not mad, out of control or bad for having these feelings. We can begin to say to ourselves, 'Yes, I do have rights and I will exercise them to help myself feel better about what I am doing and feeling.'

As our honesty grows, we can feel our alliance between our Child and Adult selves growing stronger and more able to deal with situations that previously rendered us helpless and depressed. Our victim stance will diminish as we think about what depresses us and find new ways of undertaking difficult issues. We will find a congruency between how we are inside and how we present ourselves on the outside.

WRITE IT OUT (AN ACTION PLAN)

Enough is enough. We have sat with our depression for long enough that we have worked through the main reasons for feeling so depressed. We have an understanding of how we got here and we have a picture of what we need to do to move ourselves on to reclaim our lives.

If you feel that you are not yet at this point, then don't continue until you do. Return to the first 7 days and stick with those principles until you are bored and frustrated.

For those of us who feel bored with the previous exercise, we are ready to tackle the practicalities of our life in order to shake out what we no longer require. Like panning for gold, we wash away the unnecessary debris from our life. We start by writing an action plan for change.

The reference for this action plan will come from Day 2. Look back to your initial responses when you wrote about your depression. This will give you the key to your action plan.

At this point you are simply writing out the action plan and not undertaking it. This will give you the freedom to write the perfect plan without fear or favour. Write out the perfect scenario, the ideal result and the faultless way it is carried out. Assume you are 100% right and let your imagination flow and liberate itself.

Your action plan will come in two sections, the 'Who' and the 'What'.

THE WHO

The Who is a plan to take up any issues with others who need to be confronted. Who do we confront? We need to confront anyone who we think is behaving in a way that is holding us back from beating depression. We need to be cautious when we establish this list because we must take into account how much of the 'exploitation' we feel is down to us remaining as the 'victim' and how much really is because the other person is exploiting us. We need to do all we can to purge ourselves of the victim culture until we can do no more, and then assess who needs to be confronted.

Write out the following:

- Who needs to be confronted?

This can be as simple as asking the neighbour if they can park a little to the left to help you get out of the drive more easily. It can be as big as facing your parents and explaining that as a child you were sexually abused by a relative and you feel hugely let down and angry that they kept sending you to the relative's house in spite of your protestations.

It can be as tricky as having an immediate boss who you think might try to fire you if you apply for a promotion within your company.

- How do they need to be confronted?

We must choose our method carefully because we want to get the right result so that we can beat our depression. We must be aware of what doesn't work for us. Stand-up rows often leave everyone exhausted. Calm discussion can be the best way. Sometimes having another person there helps. On occasions, mediation is the best way.

- When are they to be confronted?

Choose your timing with care. We want to get the best from ourselves and the other person. We need to be clear of our rights and sure of what our limits are – this is when we confront them.

- What result do you want from confronting them?

Envisage the perfect result before you start. Write it down if necessary. Plan it in your head. If you want to hurt some-one, that will not help you beat depression. Instead it will leave you with a guilty conscience once the initial euphoria has gone. Imagine the outcome as an adult, not a child. Think about how a great diplomat would approach the issue. The perfect result is leaving the table with our heads held high, a skip in our walk and the satisfaction that we have taken care of ourselves.

Sometimes we need to confront someone without actually `taking the problem to them. We do it this way because it's not always good for us to directly face someone we want to confront if it denies us our integrity. For instance, confronting an abusive person and receiving a verbal backlash is not always in our best interest, especially if we are depressed. We may not have enough clarity to respond in a way that protects us.

The four questions of the action plan are simply a guide to help us home in on the main cause of our pain and frustration. Not dealing with a chronic situation renders us depressed, so the questions will help us to get to the bottom of the 'cause and effect' scenario.

When we are depressed, we need to be clear and firm to ourselves who we want to confront and why. We must decide if we need to confront another or identify the historic anger and hurt. The more we can go inside ourselves and repair past damage, the clearer and stronger we feel about confronting others.

By confront, we don't mean shout and bawl our heads off. Confront means to face facts, to tackle or deal with. It means to come out from behind the sofa and sort out something we have been trying to avoid. Avoidance leads to depression. If we aren't ready to confront, then we must go back and look at why we are depressed and find our anger.

We must confront ourselves

When we try to establish who is to blame for our depression, we find that the bottom line usually sits with us. No matter how much we want to blame another person for the way we feel, we can't, except for cases of serious abuse, because we have reduced our own choices.

Lola is depressed because James 'holds her back' by not allowing her to continue with her career. Justin is depressed because his mother is still criticising him even though he is in his mid-30s. Rachael is depressed because David won't stop drinking.

We have to confront ourselves by asking what it is that we are frightened to lose if we tackle these problems. Lola is afraid of losing James's financial support; Justin is afraid of losing his mother's approval; Rachael is frightened of being on her own. We compromise ourselves for a so-called easy life. If we do this through choice then we are living with integrity. If we do this as a victim, we are blackmailing ourselves. If we are depressed, we have usually allowed another to get away with behaviour that we shouldn't tolerate. But it is our responsibility to change it by taking control of a situation or removing ourselves from it. This is our choice, our freedom and our path to reclaiming our life.

THE WHAT

For the 'What' we have to confront in our lives we need to look at the practical changes we can put into place, for example:

- I need to change my job
- I want to move house
- I have to change my financial circumstances
- I need a break

Before we begin we must first address who, if anyone, is holding us back from making these changes. There is usually someone of whom we think, 'If it weren't for them then I would have succeeded by now.' It can feel as if we are attached to another person by a spring that will pull us back if we try to separate ourselves from them. Or it may feel that there is too much at stake to lose, in which case we must weigh up the balancing act – lose 'it' or stay depressed. It can be that simple a choice.

Once we have clarified 'who' is holding us back, it's time to write out the action plan. A simple technique to help us prepare a strategy is to use the 'First Step First' plan. This will help us to decide how to tackle seemingly enormous changes.

In a double-page spread of your journal, write down the following:

GOAL TO BE ACHIEVED: – at the top of the left-hand page.
FIRST STEP FIRST – at the bottom of the right-hand page.

At the Goal To Be Achieved, you write just that, i.e. what you want to achieve. Underneath that you write the last thing you need to do to make it happen. Underneath that you write what needs to happen before that and so on. By the time you get to the bottom, you will have the first thing you need to put into place to get you started in reaching your goal. An example of this follows:

- GOAL TO BE ACHIEVED: I want to run a marathon
- I need to run three half-marathons
- I need to run 10 km three times a week
- I need to run 5 km three times a week
- I need to run 2 km three times a week
- I need to attend the gym three times a week
- I need to employ a trainer and get a fitness programme worked out
- I need to power-walk for one hour three times a week
- I need to start walking for 15 minutes three times a week
- FIRST STEP FIRST

When you follow this plan, you will feel less overwhelmed and more in control of your life because it allows you to get a grasp of a challenge and break it down so that you can see exactly what needs to be done first.

So, if you need to deal with a practical matter you have identified as holding you back, write out the First Step First plan with your top line being what you want to achieve.

TOMORROW WE TAKE ACTION.

DAY 13

Surrender No More – Take Action

'First ask yourself: What is the worst that can happen? Then prepare to accept it. Then proceed to improve on the worst.'

DALE CARNEGIE, AMERICAN AUTHOR, TRAINER

It's time to take action and put into place the work of the last 12 days. It's easy to put it off when we are depressed. But we must urge ourselves to move forward. We must find the courage to challenge what is holding us back. If we have done the work thoroughly, we will be ready, because we will have moved out of isolation and the 'stuck-ness' that depression fills us with.

If we can't make the move yet, we must examine our fears. We can work through the 'First Step First' plan again and take our time in simply shifting ourselves one step at a time.

WHAT IF WE CAN'T TAKE ACTION?

'Many of our fears are tissue-paper-thin, and a single courageous step would carry us clear through them.' BRENDAN FRANCIS

If we can't take action, or can't be bothered to take action, we have to look at why not. There are several reasons why this is and they are as follows.

'It's not that bad'

We have read the book and weighed up the ideas and decided that our depression is not that bad and these ideas are for someone else. If we are at this point, we are not really suffering. Or we are too afraid to do what we know is necessary to conquer it. If this is the case, we need to comfort our Child and form a plan that makes the necessary action challenging but manageable. We must step back until we are prepared.

We want a 'quick fix'

We want immediate relief and these ideas are too long and cumbersome. Depending on how long we have been depressed, we may find that we have tried quick fixes and they simply haven't worked. The most common fix I use is to tell myself that I'm overreacting when it comes to responding to another person in a way that feels horrible inside. I don't want to have to look at why I feel like that; I don't want to have to take responsibility for myself; I don't want to have to say something to someone in order to set my limits and tell them what I need. It's hard work, so the fix is to tell myself that I've got it wrong and they are acting OK. The trouble is, I compromise myself by avoiding the nitty-gritty of communicating with someone else. It's hard work for me and I don't find it easy. So I say nothing and 'grin and bear' it. This works for a short time, then I find myself becoming irritated with them and wanting to be sarcastic or shaming. I must then swallow those utterances if we are to remain friends. In turn I swallow the problem, and I feel bad about myself and eventually get depressed.

We are angry

Maybe we are so angry that we won't try to attempt someone else's suggestions. We feel patronised and loathing of anyone else trying to tell us how we feel. We are still angry and we haven't got to the pain. We have to go back and address the 'seesaw' of pain and anger, which is too high at the angry end.

Going it alone

When we are depressed the easy option is not to ask for help as we don't want other people to be involved in our life. This risks stagnation, because if we don't open our hearts to others, we stay stuck with the idea that there is something wrong with us and this leads us into isolation.

We have to take that first risky step of reaching out and asking another to be a friend, even if it's only a two-minute conversation. It's a continuous amazement to me how a short exchange with someone else can feel so profound. In being honest with a trusted colleague at the start of the day, I have turned my depression around with a short exchange by telling them exactly how I feel and having them nodding with understanding and reflecting on their own status. It's enough and it works. The secret is getting the conditions right to create the trust needed to open up.

We are sorting everyone else out

When we are depressed it is easy for us to focus on everyone else's needs and disregard our own. We can feel as if we have no value and the only worth we feel comes from helping others out. We may ignore pleas to stop, for to stop would be too painful. We may choose others who are unable to tell us to stop. We may choose to feel angry that we are not appreciated and then we can forget that we are depressed because we have the martyr stance to save us from our depression.

We are simply too depressed

If this is the case then we are not ready and we can rest up. It's not our time and we cannot push ourselves any more. Depression involves forcing ourselves to be 'happy' when we're not or 'pro-active' when we can't be. If it isn't time for us to take action then we can simply choose not to.

STOP THE BLACK & WHITE THINKING

Black-and-white thinking is common for some of us who have become very depressed. It's the 'all or nothing' scenario voicing the extremity of our feelings. For example, 'I will never get out of this mess'; 'I will never feel good again'; 'This is how my life is going to be forever'; this is the manner in which we think in our depressed moments. The struggle to beat depression just feels too hard.

The consequences of thinking like this can spiral us downwards as our thoughts tell us that the world is a bad place and that we are victims. Black-and-white thinking keeps us stuck, as we see life as a series of crises to be 'got through'. We are acting as a child with no defence and no rights. We must remain aware that we have rights and we have the power to assert them.

This mode of thinking will begin to lessen as we put right what has dented us and we feel less like a victim. There are ways to lessen black-and-white thinking.

Thinking Neutral

Thinking Neutral can enable us to feel more balanced and at ease with the world. It is about learning to accept events with a more impartial approach. With black-and-white thinking we can often feel that every event has happened just to try and get at us. But this is not reality. Events happen and people say and do things that really have no impact on us except for the way we view them.

Thinking Neutral can help us to start seeing events as clouds moving across the sky while we watch them go by. We don't get upset about what we can't change as we accept our powerlessness over events and other people. We don't raise our hopes to dizzy heights. We feel less sad as we realise that most of our gloom is about a perceived or threatened loss and rarely about something we have actually lost.

Through Neutral Thinking we can start to live with a certain detachment that enables us to watch and feel the reaction we have to life's events without getting caught up in them. In terms of the Adult/Parent/Child split, it is like an adult watching a child carefully as she plays in the park with others; the adult is attuned to the variety of emotions, reactions and tussles the child goes through without actually getting involved, making judgements or having any reaction. Unless the child is in danger, the adult watches life go on without any worry, knowing that it's just life happening.

One of the hardest but most profound feats to accomplish is letting go of our 'highs'. Viewing 'highs' as being as disruptive as 'lows' is a complex task. We are constantly bombarded with images, sounds and ideas of what will give us the 'nirvana' we all crave and it seems to arrive in money, cars, property, clothes etc. The distraction that we nurture and celebrate takes us far away from Neutral Thinking and can result in depression, because we do not receive the comfort and love that the Child part of us needs to feel warm and secure. We are too busy relying on external things to give us a temporary high. Having 'things' clutters us up and, if we are on that circuit, someone else will always have more. So we are constantly striving to succeed in material gain.

Many people say, yes, but you have to pay the bills. Yes, we have to pay the bills but if we are trying to beat our depression by working ourselves into the ground so we can buy 'highs' or constantly looking for others' approval, we have lost our own power and control. This is beyond working to pay the bills, this is obsessive working and will bring us further away from 'neutral thinking'.

Just Say STOP

A simple start to lessening black-and-white thinking is to say to ourselves, when we find our minds racing along at a hundred miles an hour, 'STOP!' We can calm our thoughts instantly with this simple technique. We may only stop the mind racing for one or two seconds to begin with, but as we practise this technique the seconds will grow. Put a big STOP! Sign on your wall and just do it every time you walk by. It's an extraordinarily simple thing but it works.

Meditation

This can be done anywhere and anytime. It is a way we can take a couple of minutes to relax and gain a little perspective:

Sit or lie down comfortably. Let your thoughts come and go for a minute. You will sense the different feelings that your thoughts engender. Now, turn your racing thoughts into a calm and still lake. Watch the lake and visualise it as quiet and placid as a mirror. You know that in the deep waters your emotions are stored. But, for the moment, you feel the calmness of the surface. If your mind starts to race, simply witness it as a third party without judgement. Notice how your feelings become calm and your stomach relaxes. As fear rises from the surface then let it float away on the surface of the lake until it becomes calm once more. Feel the beauty of the lake's surface. Feel the stillness in your soul.

This meditation need only be a few minutes long. It is a little sanctuary that's available to us any time we want. It is not meant to be an in-depth meditation but a tool to develop that will give us a bolthole in the middle of the day, when we are sitting

on the tube or on the loo when we have taken a break from
a stressful meeting. It's one of those things that gets better
the more we practise.

There are many fantastic books and tapes available to us
for all types of meditation. There are complete programmes
devoted to teaching us how to integrate meditation into our
lives and using it as a tool for combating stress. Whether we
invest in one of these or use a simple technique like the one
above, we will benefit by these techniques. Find a technique
that works for you, and it will quieten your racing mind and
help to stop your black-and-white thinking.

Whatever our preference, we must put in place a change
in our thinking in order that we take on new thoughts. 'Racing
thoughts' is an epidemic for those of us who are depressed.
Our thinking numbs our spirit and it is important that we try
new techniques to help combat our racing minds to help forge
a space for healing. For those of us who have suffered from
depression for a long time, we will probably always be
susceptible to depression, and employing meditation will help
us to change our habits to keep depression at bay. At its best,
meditation can help us reach a state of joy that we never
knew was possible.

DAY 14
Change The Way You See It

'A pessimist sees the difficulty in every opportunity; an optimist sees the opportunity in every difficulty.'

SIR WINSTON CHURCHILL (1874–1965)

When we are depressed we tend to see the negative side of a situation. We see the glass as half empty instead of half full. We have learned to do this over a period of time. When we are depressed we often hear others tell us that it is not that bad, they can't see what the problem is or that we are making a mountain out of a molehill. We can feel angry and patronised. How is it that they see it another way yet we are both looking at the same thing? It's because their information is filtered through a different pattern and a dissimilar history to us. They have been taught in a different manner to us.

But this is all learned. We are not 'born depressed'. We can change the way we see life and events and it is frighteningly simple. It is so simple it may put you off trying it out! But I urge you to try this technique and see for yourself; once you get a positive result you can try it with anything. Only when you get to this last stage in beating depression can you begin to grasp the idea that things can change, because you will have seen and felt changes take place already.

When you face a scenario in which you can only see gloom or disaster, find the antidote. There is an antidote to every situation in our life and we can find it. We may not like or want the antidote but that doesn't mean there isn't one. There is an upside to every drama we face.

Here are some examples:

Someone stole my mobile phone

On the surface, nothing good could come from this. However, a phone can be blocked and a new one acquired with the financial damage being minimal. This will teach us to take better care of our belongings in case someone tries it again. It could have been so much worse if our wallet and credit cards were taken with a sum of cash, or worse still, a cherished item. Losing a phone might mean we lose many numbers that were stored on it. However, it is sometimes a good day to have a 'clear out' and that includes numbers of people we never really wanted to call again. Those that count will make contact.

I can't get ahead in my career

It can feel like a dead end when we can't move forward in our career. However, it may be a time to step back and stop pushing. If nothing is coming our way it could be because it's just not the right time. When we try and force change when it's not the right time we end up feeling completely dejected. The upside of this scenario is to seize the opportunity to establish what we really want to do rather than what we think we should do. If you are unclear about what you want to do then there is a great saying that goes, 'Identify your obsession, make it your profession.' This is better advice than any career counsellor I have ever encountered.

I have nothing to wear

Most of us do have something to wear. In fact, we often have so much to wear that we have too much choice and this can leave us in despair. What we often mean is that we don't have anything new to wear. We also feel that our image depends on what we wear. This is a symptom of our society and we can choose to kowtow to that indicator or we can choose not to be influenced by it. Indeed, it is incredibly therapeutic to challenge the view that we have nothing to wear because it helps us to keep in check that desperate side of us that needs 'stuff' in order to help us feel better.

I can't find a partner

Trying to find a partner can be a way of wanting to get someone else to help us feel better about ourselves. We cannot conduct an adult, loving relationship when we are deprived of self-nurture and affection. Being single gives us a great opportunity to help ourselves to grow up and finish our childhood. We should revel in our time alone. We can make huge strides in taking advantage of not being in a relationship. Many of us find that sorting ourselves out works better when we are single because we don't have to give to another and compromise ourselves. We can remind ourselves of this daily with a journal entry, Post-it note or by talking to another. Help is also at hand by attending Co-Dependants Anonymous, which deals with the difficulties we encounter in relationships. Knowing we have choices gives us hope and can liberate us from the fantasy that finding a partner will solve our problems.

I'm fat

Being overweight does not render us bad or unlovable. There are many people who are overweight but not depressed. The upside is that we have choices. No one is forcing us to be overweight. Being overweight is often due to feeling depressed and having little self-respect. This might be because we have not given enough psychological nurturing to ourselves. We can turn this situation around by changing the message we give ourselves. We can take time out from trying to look better for other people and concentrate more on feeling better for us.

FIND YOUR JUICE

There is one thing that 'gets' us; that 'does it' for us. We have to find it – this is our Juice. Everyone has something that fills them with joy, freedom and fun. When we are depressed we think this means everyone except us. We must consider this our arrogance. We are not aliens and we do not work differently to everyone else. We can find our Juice.

Our Juice is the one thing we do that brushes away the cobwebs. It is the action that holds a line to our soul, our spirit, our essence, our Child. It is the thing we do that puts the fun back into our lives. It is something that fulfils us like no other. We have to find it and make sure we can carry it out regularly so that we feel completely satisfied afterwards.

It may seem like a small thing, and when we are depressed we can easily brush it aside as a trivial exercise or a waste of time. But we have to change the way we think about our Juice and actively employ it for our good. Our Juice may change as we grow older but there will always be something that does the job – however simple. For example:

- Sue has found it through weeding. After she has weeded she feels reconnected, rejuvenated and whole.
- Barbara loves to crochet. She feels great when she is quietly working on her next assignment.
- Sally loves to make crafts projects with her children.
- Harry's Juice is to go sailing. When he's been out in his dinghy, he comes back a new man.
- Linda is never happier than when she is cooking a great meal for her boyfriend.
- Susan is at one with the world when she goes on a picnic – whatever the weather.
- Frances loves to clear a room up and throw away at least 10% of it.
- I like to exercise. After a session at the gym, I come home feeling as if I have got life in perspective.

Find your Juice, exploit it, and make it help you beat depression and reclaim your life.

THINGS THAT WILL COME OUT OF THESE 14 DAYS:

1 We will no longer run our life as a child in an adult world. We are now ruled by our wisdom and set free, to play and enjoy life, by our emotions.

2 We no longer feel there is a judge and jury waiting outside our front door to criticise us. We will look left and right and see they have gone.

3 We can let go of what others do and how they behave. The effect that others have on us has lessened and we don't feel the need to control them.

4 We will cry more easily and be less burdened with a feeling of 'stuck-ness'. We will be able to let go of grief as it arises. This leaves us feeling more cleansed than ever before, as we will not let ourselves become blocked and angry.

5 We need less materially because we are not as starved emotionally.

6 We relish being different from others and we like to stand back from the herd. We know that standing alone can be scary because we are saying that we don't want to be like everyone else. We want people to like us as we are, but we don't need their support to feel OK because we have developed the support systems for ourselves by identifying our Adult, our Child and our Higher Power. We have built bridges to others that can help us.

7 We feel powerful because we know that we can stop toxic thinking by replacing an old critical message with a new one. We know how effective this is, and we can even put an exercise in place today and know that we will feel different and more accepting by tomorrow.

8 We trust ourselves more as we notice how we feel more quickly. We develop the link between our intellect and our emotions until we can track and anticipate how we are going to react to people and events.

9 We start to realise our potential and we feel ourselves growing tall as we turn corners we would previously have avoided, say things we

have never felt the courage to say before, and take on ventures that would previously have felled us at the first hurdle.

10 We have reached an integrity that we never thought was possible. This integrity exposes itself in the way we feel about our world; we know our limits, we understand our choices, we know the rules we might break by choice, we are aware of our motives and we are conscience of how we affect others. We use our power, but never to abuse another. We stretch ourselves for our own satisfaction. We acknowledge the laws but we take action as we see fit for ourselves. We love life. We plan but we don't project. We feel a sense of congruence between how we feel and how we present ourselves to the world.

WE HAVE COME HOME.

Resources

SANE

Provides information and emotional support to those experiencing mental health problems, their families and carers through SANELINE.
0845 767 8000 (12 noon to 2 a.m.)
http://www.sane.org.uk

MIND

The MindinfoLine offers thousands of callers confidential help on a range of mental health issues. MIND also provide a special legal service to the public, lawyers and mental health workers.
0845 766 0163 (Mon–Fri, 9.15 a.m. to 4.45 p.m.)
Granta House, 15–19 Broadway, London E15 4BQ   www.mind.org.uk

RETHINK

Rethink runs more than 300 services around England, Wales and Northern Ireland, which give practical support for around 7,500 people every day.
Rethink general enquiries:
0845 456 0455 or email
info@rethink.org
National advice line: 020 8974 6814 (Mon–Fri, 10 a.m. to 3 p.m.)
or email advice@rethink.org
http://www.rethink.org/services/

STEADY

Steady is a self-management training programme for young people with the mental health diagnosis of bipolar disorder (manic depression) or extreme mood swings. The Steady training course is open to residents of the British Isles aged 18 to 25 years old.
Address: Castle Works,
21 St George's Rd, London SE1 6ES
Tel: 020 7793 2600   Email:
Steady@mdf.org.uk

THE MENTAL HEALTH FOUNDATION

The biggest, most comprehensive website on mental health in the UK. The site is run by the Mental Health Foundation, the leading UK charity working in mental health and learning disabilities.
The Mental Health Foundation,
83 Victoria Street, London SW1H 0HW.
Tel: 020 7802 0300 Fax: 020 7802 0301
Email. mhf@mhf.org.uk
http://www.mentalhealth.org.uk/

THE MANIC DEPRESSION FELLOWSHIP

Produces information and advice specifically related to manic depression or bipolar disorder.
Castle Works, 21 St Georges Road, London SE1 6ES
National Advice Line 0208 7793 2600
Scotland Advice Line 0141 400 1867
Wales Advice Line 01633 244 244
(Mon–Thurs, 9 a.m. to 4 p.m., Fri, 9 a.m. to 5 p.m.)
http://www.mdf.org.uk/

STAND

Defeatdepression.org is dedicated
to pursuing the advancement of
information and support for all those
suffering from stress, anxiety or
depression. It offers cutting-edge
information and support.
http://www.defeatdepression.org

ADDICTION RECOVERY FOUNDATION

The Addiction Recovery Foundation
is a UK-based charity dedicated to
providing current information on
the treatment and recovery from
addictions and dependencies.
Addiction Recovery Foundation,
122A Wilton Road, London SW1V 1JZ
Tel: 020 7233 5333 Fax: 020 7233 8123
http://www.addictiontoday.co.uk/

AWARE

Provides information and support
to people affected by depression
in Ireland and Northern Ireland.
72 Lower Leeson Street,
Dublin 2, Republic of Ireland
(01) 6766166 (Every day, 10 a.m.
to 10 p.m.)

THE ASSOCIATION OF
POST-NATAL ILLNESS

Information on post-natal
depression, and will put mothers
affected by post-natal depression
in touch with others who have
had similar experiences.
145 Dawes Rd, Fulham,
London SW6 7EB
020 7386 0868

THE BRITISH ASSOCIATION
FOR COUNSELLING

Provides information and advice on
all matters related to counselling. They
can also send you a list of accredited
counsellors in your local area.
1 Regent Place, Rugby,
Warwickshire CV21 2PJ
01788 550 899 (8.45 a.m. to 4.45 p.m.)
www.bac.co.uk

THE BRITISH ASSOCIATION FOR
BEHAVIOURAL AND COGNITIVE
PSYCHOTHERAPIES

Will provide a directory of registered
therapists for £2.00 including postage.
PO Box 9, Accrington, BB5 2GD.
Tel/fax: 01254 875277

CALM

Helpline for young men who
are depressed or suicidal.
0800 585858 (Every day, 5 p.m. to 3 a.m.)

CARERS LINE

Helpline providing advice and
information for carers on any issue
0808 808 7777 (Mon–Fri, 10 a.m.
to 12 noon, 2 p.m. to 4 p.m.)

CRUSE Bereavement Care

Information and advice for
people who are bereaved.
Cruse House, 126 Sheen Road,
Richmond, Surrey TW9 1UR
020 8940 4818 (Helpline &
information line, Mon–Fri,
9.30 a.m. to 5 p.m.)
www.crusebereavementcare.org.uk

HEALTH INFORMATION SERVICE

Information on all health-
related subjects including
where to get treatment.
0800 665 544 (Mon–Fri, 9 a.m. to 5 p.m.
(may vary according to locality)

LESBIAN AND GAY
BEREAVEMENT PROJECT

Offers support and counselling
for bereavement and AIDS.
Unitarian Rooms, Hoop Lane,
London NW11 ORL
020 8455 8894 200

MEDICATION AND DRUGS HELPLINE

Confidential information about
prescription drugs from trained
medical professionals.
020 7919 2999 (Mon–Fri, 11 a.m.
to 5 p.m.)

NATIONAL PHOBICS SOCIETY

Helpline for people affected
by anxiety, phobias, compulsive
disorders, or panic attacks.
0161 227 9898
(Mon–Fri, 10.30 a.m. to 4 p.m.)

PACE

Counselling, mental health
advocacy and group work
for lesbians and gay men.
020 7697 0017
(Mon–Thurs, 10 a.m. to 9 p.m.)

PARENTLINE

Helpline and information
for parents in distress.
8800 2222
(Mon–Fri, 9 a.m. to 9 p.m.)

RELATE NATIONAL OFFICE

Offers counselling on relationship
problems for couples or individuals.
Herbert Gray College, Little Church
Street, Rugby CV21 3AP
01788 573 241

ROYAL COLLEGE OF PSYCHIATRISTS

Offers information about
mental illness.
17 Belgrave Square,
London SW1X 8PG
020 7235 2351

S.A.D. ASSOCIATION

Provides information and advice
on seasonal affective disorder.
PO Box 989, Steyning,
West Sussex BN44 3HG

THE SAMARITANS

Offer confidential emotional
support to any person who is
suicidal or despairing.
46 Marshall Street, London W1V 1LR
08457 90 90 90 (24 hours, every day)

SCOTTISH ASSOCIATION
FOR MENTAL HEALTH

Support, information and advice
on various aspects of mental health.
Cumbrie House, 15 Carlton Court,
Glasgow G5 9JP 0141 568 7000

YOUNG MINDS PARENTS
INFORMATION LINE

Helpline offering information
and support on young peoples'
mental health for parents.
0800 0182138 (Mon & Fri, 10 a.m. to 1 p.m.,
Tues, Wed & Thurs, 9 a.m. to 4 p.m.)

DEPRESSION ALLIANCE

Depression Alliance is a UK charity offering help to people with depression, run by sufferers themselves. The website contains information about the symptoms of depression, treatments for depression, as well as Depression Alliance campaigns and local groups. National Office: Depression Alliance, 35 Westminster Bridge Road, London SE1 7JB
Tel: 0207 633 0557
Fax: 0207 633 0559
www.depressionalliance.org

THE BRITISH ACUPUNCTURE COUNCIL

The UK's main regulatory body for the practice of acupuncture by over 2200 professionally qualified acupuncturists.
63 Jeddo Road, London, W12 9HQ
020 8735 0400
www.acupuncture.org

12-STEP FELLOWSHIPS

ALCOHOLICS ANONYMOUS (AA)

AA is designed for those who have a drinking problem and wish to give up. Approx. 3,000 UK groups. GSO: PO Box l, Stonebow House, Stonebow, York, YO1 7NJ
Information, literature and contacts, also for Europe: 01904 644026
London: 020 7833 0022 (10 a.m. to 10 p.m. Answer phone other times)
www.alcoholics-anonymous.org

AL-ANON

This is the place for those people who are affected by another person's drinking. Family Groups UK & Eire: 61 Great Dover Street, London SE1 4YF
Information and details of group meetings: 020 7403 0888
(24-hour confidential helpline)
www.al-anon.org

ADULT CHILDREN OF ALCOHOLICS AND DYSFUNCTIONAL FAMILIES

These groups are for adults raised in alcoholic or dysfunctional families and still suffer the implications but wish to recover.
PO Box 1576, London SW3 1AZ
07071 781899
www.adultchildren.org

CO-DEPENDANTS ANONYMOUS

For those people who cannot maintain a healthy relationship. Information: SAE to Asburnham Community Centre, Tetcott Road, Chelsea, London SW10 0SH
020 7376 8191
www.ourcoda.org

NARCOTICS ANONYMOUS

For people addicted to narcotics.
UK Service Office, PO Box 1980,
London N19 3LS
Literature listings, information:
020 7251 4007
Helpline (10 a.m. to 10 p.m.
weekdays; weekend redirect):
020 7730 0009
Recorded meeting list for London:
020 7281 9933
www.wsoinc.com

FAMILIES ANONYMOUS

For relatives and friends of those
with drug problems. Literature given.
Approx 50 UK groups.
Doddington & Rollo Community
Association, Charlotte Despard
Avenue, Battersea, London SW11
020 7498 4680
www.famanon.org

OVEREATERS ANONYMOUS

For anyone who has a problem with
food, including anorexics. 140 groups
in the UK. Tel: 07000 784985
(national), 01426 984674 (London)
http://overeaters.org

SEX ADDICTS ANONYMOUS

For those who need to engage
in obsessive sex or sexual activity.
BCM, Box 1457, London WC1N 3XX.
London SAA Intergroup, meetings
information and callback answer
phone: 020 8442 7278
www.saa-recovery.org

GAMBLERS ANONYMOUS

For those who cannot stop gambling.
http://gamblersanonymous.org

WORKAHOLICS ANONYMOUS

For those who find work is
controlling their lives.
PO Box 11466, London SW1V 2ZQ
Contact Celia on 01993 878220
& 020 7834 5736 or
David on 01895 811011

'This empowering read leads you away from fog where eerie shadows and distant growls taunt to a place called home with familiar shapes and friendly voices.'

SALLY COOKE

'In spite of the subject matter the sheer enthusiasm, understanding and practical advice conveyed by the author who has obviously "been through the mill" came shining through and provided me with an IMMEDIATE lift and a will to action the advice given.'

BRIAN CROSS

'This book is a quick shot of empathy and sound advice for the days when you need it most. Alexandra Massey puts depression in perspective without downplaying its crushing effects. The good news is, you don't have to feel crushed anymore. I've tried all the suggestions in this book and have been amazed at how quickly they could bring relief at the worst of times.'

JANE WANGER